Return to Human: How Modern Medicine, the Media, and the Mundane Have Destroyed our Health and How to Move Back Towards Optimal Health

D1563204

Jorge Roman Lopez

Memento mori

.

CONTENTS

FOREWORD BY DR. JOEL GOULD

The foundation of every state is the education of its youth.
- Diogenes

The quote above is one from Diogenes, also known as "Diogenes the Cynic", a Greek philosopher born in 404 BC. Diogenes was known for revolting against social norms and bucking the accepted trends and behaviors in many areas of society he felt were corrupt. This "cynical" concept is more relevant than ever in the modern world. We are stuck in the past with a failing medical paradigm, despite technology and social norms changing more quickly than ever before.

It's interesting to see how the word "cynic" has evolved to be something negative, instead of describing an interest in questioning norms of the times for the betterment of mankind, and an open-minded curiosity of life.

Over the years, we have taken many wrong turns with our health and how we care for our biological bodies. The results are plain to see: chronic inflammatory health issues, obesity, mental health issues, and a weakened immune system. As technology connects us all, information—right or wrong, helpful or not—is easily and quickly disseminated. The internet, digital media, and social platforms share information almost instantly and effortlessly. But who do we listen to, and who do we trust? Who deserves our time in such a busy world of so many screeching voices competing for attention?

We need clear new voices, from every generation of society, but from our youth, especially, as they are literally the future of this planet. I have been fearful of our new world of young social media influencers and the focus on building a brand and followers as the currency. The influencers, however, have focused on the "how", and don't seem to have a clear "why" they want to influence anyone anyway.

Jorge Roman is one of those new voices that has a powerful why, and a vision. We need the voices of the next generation to clearly see the predicament we are in when it comes to our bodies, our future health, and the health of the planet. There is a need for a revolution and excitement, and willingness for our young people to come together, and unite against the dangers of globalization, control of our healthcare, and food chain.

Jorge, thank you for listening to the wise voices of the scientists who are sharing truth, without bias and conflicts of interest. Thank you for becoming fascinated with health, and wellness. It's you, and the younger generation that has been, and will continue to be the most impacted by the damage of this current failed medical paradigm. Build strong connections with your compatriots and collaborate to share the truth about natural and organic health. Your voice in youth is strong, unwavering, and credible. Continue to question accepted science and use common sense to evaluate what you see.

Return to Human is an accessible, engaging, and a highly topical view of what's gone wrong with modern healthcare, and humanity. Read it, investigate its contents, adapt as needed with its recommendations, and share it with anyone open to a different view of health. This book, simply and adeptly put together, is a powerful snapshot in time of the world we are living in as it transforms in front of our eyes. *Return to Human* is a powerful tool for those who want to quickly and easily improve their health.

Cynicism can be a good thing, if it's followed up with investigation, and an open-minded curiosity to learn and discover. Bucking accepted trends that are not well supported by evidence is the kind of uprising we need. Cynicism may sound negative, but information, shared with a strong, confident voice is the tool that shapes the future generations knowledge. It's heartening to see the voice of a young and thoughtful health and wellness expert begin to grow.

Our state has failed us, and the education it is providing its citizens with is fatally flawed and beginning to crumble away in front of our eyes. In this book you will find an understanding of science, appropriate research, and a clear message of common sense.

Thank you, Jorge, for your positive view of cynicism. It's what the world needs to return to human.

PREFACE

I sat in my doctor's office a few weeks before my sophomore year. I had recently decided to compete again after my first summer off in *years*. That meant, I had to get my sports physical done. So, there I was making light conversation while my doctor prodded my genitals and whacked my knee with a hammer. Everything was going smoothly. Then, it was time for the uncomfortable questions. You know, the *fun* questions: "*Are you sexually active? If so, are you wearing a condom? Have you been tested for STIs? Do you drink alcohol? Drugs?*" Then came a question which felt strangely unfamiliar—not because I had never been asked it, but because, for the first time, every fiber of my being wanted to blurt out: *Yes.*

"*Any thoughts of suicide?*"

My mouth dried up. I burst out crying. I couldn't even answer the damn question. What the hell was wrong with me? For a split-second I looked up to see my doctor wide-eyed, caught off guard just as I was. When I finally managed to calm down, I told her it wasn't serious—I was just having a bad day. I told her to not tell my mom, who was patiently sitting in the waiting room. Her lip stiffened and the sides of her mouth curved downward, but she said, *"Ok"*. I saw my doctor reach for a pen and a sticky note. Knowing that I was heading off to college soon, she wrote down an email, a phone number, and a name. *"Please. Don't hesitate to call or email her. She's a great therapist."*

I walked out of the room. Unable to hide the emotional hailstorm which had hit me moments ago, my mom, as any other good mom, immediately began to investigate. That was a fun conversation.

"What happened?! Are you ok?"

"Yes, mom"

"Are you sure you're ok?"

"Yes, mom. Just having a bad day. I don't know what it was"

"You know, maybe we could sit down with your dad and…"

"Absolutely not."

I made it through a couple more weeks of loving scrutiny before it was finally time to go back to school. What I considered to be a wildly random emotional outburst seemed to be just that—at least, for a few weeks. Then, it slowly began to resurface, each time with a vengeance. I guess Freud was right.

When I got to school, I decided to enroll in a class called philosophy of religion. A few weeks into the semester, we started to read "A Confession" by Leo Tolstoy. If you haven't read the book, it outlines Tolstoy's thought process as he pondered taking his own life. As I read the book, it was as if *I had written it.* Don't get me wrong, I'm not suggesting my own writing is as good as Tolstoy's. It just seemed to me that my own thoughts were closely mirrored in his writing. In contemplating suicide, my mind followed a similar logic as his. And the strange part was—it did, in fact, feel *logical*. It went a little something like this: *Life is filled with suffering and ends in death. I'm taking up limited space, food, and oxygen. I do not deserve the things I have. If I die, the world will keep spinning as if nothing happened. I don't owe anyone anything—I did not choose to be born. If I die, I will feel no more pain.* Anyone with any sense can probably agree that most, if not all, of those statements are true. Here was the problem: that's *all* I could see. Any other interpretations of life didn't feel emotionally, nor logically, relevant. When you get in that mindset, you start to relentlessly ask yourself: *"What's the point?"* Now, to be clear, I didn't ask it like a sophomore philosophy major intellectually masturbating in front of his peers. I asked it *with all the seriousness in the world*. When I first began to ask this question, my brain came up with some half-assed answers which, for some time, kept it at bay. But, like some sort of ravenous monster, it wasn't *ever* truly satisfied. After dozens of times *really* asking myself, *"What's the point?"* I left myself no choice but to be brutally honest with myself: I had no idea. As I asked it more frequently, I came to the conclusion that *there was no point*.

As I went about my day, thoughts of ending my life rattled in my mind like a sharp stone stubbornly stuck in a shoe.

They were there—reliable—as I woke up and as I prepared for bed. They were there with every forkful of food I ate. They were there with every drive I took, nudging me to let go of the steering wheel and press my foot on the gas. Dark daydreams seeped into the most mundane activities.

What's the least painful?

The quickest?
The quietest?
No, not that one—that won't work. Too expensive.

As these thoughts increased in amplitude, I found myself at the mercy of my emotions. While this was internally true, I was very good at hiding it from most people. When I'd come back to my dorm after dinner, I'd force myself to act how I normally act. I joked around, spent some time with my friends, and then went to my room. Since I had a roommate, the pretending couldn't end just yet. After a few more forced smiles, gossip, and small talk, I turned off the lights in preparation for sleep. That's when the floodgates opened. In order to hold back uncontrollable sobbing, I'd smother my face with my pillow, stuffing it into my mouth to drown out all sound.

It was a strange sensation, sobbing like I hadn't sobbed since elementary school. I couldn't wrap my head around it. Logically speaking, I knew exactly what the next step was. Why was I crying? It was almost as if *my body* was mourning for *me*.

Needless to say, I was utterly consumed. But there was just one thing stopping me every time I got close to making the decision: *the people who cared about me*. Simply put, I didn't want to hurt them. Sounds mind-numbingly obvious, but in that state of mind, things didn't make the same sort of sense.

As more thoughts of suicide intruded my mind, the once nebulous idea of taking my own life became increasingly *clear*. But I'd always find myself at the same spot—I just couldn't do it to the people around me. Then, *eureka*—a loophole occurred to me. If I was really going to make the decision to end my life, I needed the people around me to not love me anymore. I certainly didn't want to cause more pain than necessary. By no means was this a conscious thought at the time. It was only after about a year of reflection that I realized it—but I believe I knew it subconsciously. And I acted accordingly.

I disguised my subconscious desire to push everyone away as words soaked in hatred and arguments which were totally unnecessary and unfounded. In a twisted sense, I succeeded. I managed to destroy some friendships, alienate myself, and paint myself in a negative light so that I could do what I set out to do.

Fortunately, I didn't get to everyone. I had a few amazing people in my life who, no matter how much I hurt, just wouldn't let me go.

And that was the turning point. When I realized they wouldn't *ever* let go, I knew I couldn't *ever* leave a permanent hole in the fabric of their lives. Without them, I would have likely become just another number added to the growing suicide statistics this past year.

So, I realized that my friends and family weren't going anywhere. Ultimately, I decided: *I no longer give myself the option of ending my life.*

If there was one thing I learned from being an athlete for 10 years, it was discipline—when I committed to doing something *I did it*. So, I committed myself to understanding why I felt and thought the way I did—no matter where I had to look. As I searched for answers, I left no stone unturned and no quack unattended—I listened to *everyone* who had something to say about treating depression and living a life worth living (even though some of the advice was useless, at best). I investigated the physical stuff: the microbiome, diet, supplements, light exposure, movement, and sleep. I looked into the mental stuff: cognitive behavioral therapy, meditation, positive affirmations, journaling, compassionate inquiry, and beyond.

Coming from a long lineage of fiery tempers and stubbornness, I realized that I needed to be the one to break that tradition if I was really going to make a change. I opened my mind to the fact that I had *no idea what I was doing.* For the most part, I found that to be, at least somewhat, true. I learned the power of shutting my ego up and just *listening*—to everyone and everything.

But what does this story have to do with anything? Ever since I was little, I could barely look someone in the eye, much less give a school presentation without my heart racing, my throat closing up, and my palms dripping with sweat. So, why on Earth would I share this personal story with you? It has to do with the main reason I wrote this book. We're at a point in history where a lack of transparency is causing absolute mayhem. To say that we're as polarized as ever before would be an understatement. Although the violent clashing of opposing ideas has always been a trademark of humanity, the modern world has lit this trait on fire. You tune into your favorite news channel because you know they'll tell you exactly what you want to hear: a one-sided story which makes you feel better about yourself by belittling and ridiculing "the other side". Because they're the dumb ones... right? Social media algorithms have now been designed to fill your feed with abrasive, emotionally loaded clickbait, which accomplishes a similar task as the news. These echo chambers of virtual reality are boosting our egos and driving division at the expense of the truth. Unfortunately, during the pandemic, it has become increasingly obvious that our politicians and even some health professionals have been fueling this phenomenon as well.

So, to be ultimately vulnerable with you about a deeply personal story is to set an important precedent. In a world of misinformation and half-truths, it's about time we start receiving the whole truth, no matter how ugly it might seem and how uncomfortable it might be. At a time when we have near-unlimited information at our fingertips, I hope we can start looking at all sides of a story rather than retweeting vitriol to make ourselves feel better. As you'll learn throughout this book, this message isn't coming from me standing on a gold-plated pedestal with a glimmering halo around my head. I was guilty of doing what I've just described to you, especially at the beginning of the pandemic. In fact, it is precisely *because* I fell prey to that behavior that I know just how much damage it causes. Therefore, I have made a commitment to myself, and to you, to be as objective as I can be throughout this book.

To tell you the truth, when I first started writing, I thought the solution to all of our health problems was either: one, to be found in the depths of PubMed—a hidden gold mine of dusty, old scientific papers just waiting to be found; or two, to reclaim our health by living exactly like our ancestors, relinquish all worldly belongings, buy a few goats and chickens and live in the countryside—you know, the typical naturalistic fallacy which argues that if something exists in nature it must be good for you, and all modern things are *bad*. Unfortunately, I did not, and have not, found either to be the source of ultimate truth.

The pandemic has made this clear as day. We've all heard wild, unsubstantiated claims by ancestral health *and* conventional medicine advocates alike. The former has mostly been guilty of claiming things like all vaccines are dangerous, but herbs will cure cancer—while providing no solid evidence. The latter has made claims like, *"There's nothing you can do to prevent a severe case of COVID-19 but wash your hands, pour bleach on your groceries, and put 4 masks on,"* while ignoring data which is inconvenient to their beliefs. Having personally experienced the consequences of dogmatic, black-or-white thinking, I forced myself to stay centered.

So, in a COVID-19 world plagued by dietary, lifestyle, and scientific dogma, I set out to let go of these biases as much as possible. I listened to *as many experts* as I could—not just the ones CNN or FOX news told me to listen to. From *"COVID is 5G"* and *"This virus was made in a lab"* to *"COVID kills everything it touches",* I entertained it *all.* Interesting that the lab leak hypothesis, which was considered conspiracy and taboo, is now widely considered to be a possibility. Shoutout to the few brave scientists who risked their careers in a hypersensitive, cancel-culture world, where discussing real science which is not *"the science"* is considered dangerous quackery. More on my definition of *"the science"* later.

By using a healthy dose of common sense, skepticism, and scientific evidence, I began putting together many different streams of information to get as close as I possibly could to the truth.

The purpose of this book is two-fold. First, I'll be sharing my journey in learning to learn: being skeptical, open to ideas which made me uncomfortable, and ultimately staying centered in search of the truth in a world which rewards snarky social media posts and tweets filled with rage. The first component feeds into the second piece of the purpose: what environmental and lifestyle factors are making people more susceptible to a severe case of COVID-19? And how can we support our health at a time when much of the world feels totally disempowered? Now you may think to yourself, as I often do, *"How the hell can a 20-year-old dude—who doesn't even know what he wants for dinner—even begin answering such a complex question?"* Good point—I ask myself that question all the time. I won't pretend to be smarter than the thousands of researchers worldwide who dedicate their lives to answering these questions.

However, here's why I'm crazy enough to believe I can do it: one, I have listened to and read the perspectives of thousands of researchers and health professionals who *are* experts in their fields; and two, doctors and researchers often *specialize*. Now, specialization isn't necessarily a bad thing, but it comes with severe limitations. Think of a researcher investigating the link between vitamin D status and the severity of COVID-19. As you'll find out later in this book, there's an undeniable link between these two. However, it's not everything. Having a proper vitamin D status supports healthy immunity, but it's far from the *only*, or the most important thing which contributes to a healthy and resilient body.

What's been missing is a synthesis of *all* the research, rather than just a few pieces of the puzzle that make the headlines. No one has put together strong, comprehensive evidence to not only dramatically reduce the risk of a severe COVID-19 case, but also reduce the risk of developing virtually *all chronic diseases*! That's about to change with this book.

By merely listening to a select few doctors and researchers featured on the nightly news, it would appear that whether or not you get a severe case of COVID-19 is *basically up to chance. Sure, there may be a few things you can do to be healthier, but it's pretty much Russian Roulette,* the common narrative goes. After expanding my sources of information beyond that which is readily available, I've learned that this doesn't seem to be the case *at all.* Now, that's not to say there isn't some "random" individual variability that influences how we respond when we get infected. This variability could very well *not* be in our power to change. It would be incredibly arrogant and dishonest to say that if you do everything in this book, you will be immune to disease––but that's not the point of this book at all. The point is: let's discover what true health actually means; and why not do *everything in your power* to make your body as resilient and healthy as possible, especially with so much uncertainty in the world, new variants coming out, and the real risk of future pandemics?

If you're currently thinking to yourself, *"But healthy people HAVE died from COVID-19 you insensitive bastard! They were jacked CrossFit dudes who worked out 3 hours a day and did intermittent fasting for 18 hours a day!".* I urge you to reconsider what health truly means and be open to the possibility that our perception of health is wildly distorted. We live in a world where health means either: the absence of disease, or a six-pack. We live in a world where disease has been normalized. 6 in 10 American adults have at least one chronic disease, while over 50% of children suffer from health conditions.

Does this mean that 4 in 10 adults and less than 50% of children are actually *healthy*? *Nope*. It's not just me saying this. In fact, the World Health Organization defines true health as, "*...a state of complete physical, mental and social well-being and not merely the absence of disease or infirmity,*"[1]. So, just because someone is *not* diagnosed with an illness does NOT mean one is optimally healthy, contrary to the eye-catching, fear-mongering news headlines. Additionally, although a six pack is often a great proxy for health, it does not necessarily mean optimal health either (explained further in chapter 9)

Before we get into the meat of this book, let me first set the scene with a modern look into our evolutionary past to begin to answer what health truly means.

P.S. I was told that it would be a good idea to add a little disclaimer: as you've already seen, some foul language was used in the making of this book, but hopefully not enough to detract from the content!

CHAPTER 1: FROM ZEBRAS TO PIZZA– –HOW DID WE GET HERE?

Although I wish I could wow you with breathtaking experiences I had when visiting hunter-gatherer populations around the world, I don't have them (yet). Unfortunately, I don't yet have a personal story about roaming the plains of Africa wearing only fur skin on my genitals. I don't yet have a firsthand account of eating raw meat with an indigenous tribe. I also don't have an unbelievable, party-worthy story to tell about a near-death experience where I escaped the jaws of a ravenous 14-foot alligator. Instead, I have many hours of reading and listening to firsthand accounts of those who *have* had those experiences, as well as reading scientific research about modern hunter-gatherer populations.

So, with all of my ignorance, let's take a mental voyage to the home of one of the last few hunter-gatherer populations on Earth: the Hadza people. Picture a vast landscape undisturbed by power lines, industry, cellphone towers, and cars. Now imagine a group of young, lean Hadza men waking up to the sunrise. They stretch and prepare for the day, retrieving their bows and arrows for the day's hunt. With plants making up only a tiny fraction of their diet during the dry season, they rely primarily on meat to survive[2]. They walk for miles, finally settling at a watering hole, waiting patiently, bows and arrows at the ready. With endurance and patience unknown to most of us laptop dwellers, they often spend entire nights by a watering hole, waiting for a thirsty animal to approach. When they finally catch a break, a zebra becomes the target (this was years ago—reportedly, they can now only hunt small animals)[3]. Once they've downed the animal, it is butchered, allowing each man to carry a leg on their back for miles with the bright sun beating on their faces. Once they get back to camp, they pair the meat with some tubers and call it a night. After such a satisfying meal, the men curl up under a tree to doze off under the dim light of the stars and the moon.

This is a scene remarkably alien to many of us who may spend entire nights waiting—not for a kill at a watering hole—but rather scrolling through social media waiting for a like. The Hadza's lives give us a rare glimpse into the lives our ancestors led thousands of years ago before the agricultural and industrial revolutions.

I hope you're not thinking to yourself, "*Oh great. Another 'Back to Nature' zealot. I bet he thinks modern medicine doesn't even work or something. I bet he's an anti-vaxer.*" But if you are, I promise you that's the furthest thing from the truth. I have gotten some of those labels thrown at me. However, I must admit that I can understand where those intellectually lazy labels come from. I understand our inherent Us vs

Them mentality—the need to label someone into a neat group to make it easier on our small, monkey brains—it's been done throughout this whole pandemic. As you read on, however, I hope you'll learn that I seek to take the best from many, often opposing viewpoints, to understand human health. The Hadza allow me to do just that.

First, let me admit something: the *average* life expectancy of the Hadza is low—in the 30s[4]. *It's settled--that means the modern lifestyle is good and hunter-gatherer lifestyles are dangerous! Ha, take that paleo dieters!*

Not so fast. The *modal* age at death—the age when most deaths occur—tells a different story. The modal age at death for the Hadza and the U.S. seems to be in the late 70s and mid-80s, respectively. Anyone who's gone through elementary or middle school math understands the effect of outliers on the average. In the case of the Hadza, the outliers come from high infant mortality, bringing the average down and making it appear as if the Hadza live nasty, short lives. That's not the case *at all*, as evidenced by the *modal* age at death which is *not* affected by outliers. But what *really* interests me about the Hadza is not their lifespan, but rather their *healthspan*. Compared to industrialized nations, they have a low incidence of chronic disease which cannot be explained by merely *not living long enough to develop chronic disease*. In fact, in the scientific literature, these modern hunter-gatherers have been referred to as "Models in Public Health" with low rates of obesity, metabolic disease, and cardiovascular disease[5]. In other words, if the Hadza make it past childbirth, they are *significantly* less likely to suffer from the chronic diseases which plague first-world nations.

Now, let's compare the Hadza lifestyle with

your modern average Joe in the United States. Joe was born in a busy urban hospital via c-section. As he grew up, he developed asthma, dermatitis, gastrointestinal conditions, and allergies to kiwis and peanuts. Fast forward to life after college and Joe is now working a comfortable desk job with a wonderful view of an artificially created pond. Every morning, Joe wakes up with his sheets on the floor—a result of hours of late-night tossing and turning. With cortisol abruptly shooting through his veins, he groans and turns over to a blaring alarm clock and hits snooze. He inhales deeply, gets dressed, puts his phone in his pocket, and heads downstairs for instant coffee, a doughnut, and a statin for his cholesterol. He drives an hour to work, walks in, and sets his belongings on his desk. Joe then sits down to prepare for a busy day of phone calls, emails, and meetings under the flickering LEDs. Around noon, he gets hungry and grabs a plain bagel with some cream cheese. After hours of mindlessly snacking on pretzels, taking calls, and staring at screens, the clock finally reaches the glorious time of 5 pm. Joe gets his things, stretches his legs for the first time since the morning, and drives home. He arrives, has some pizza, and sits down in front of a bright TV screen. It is now 10:30 pm and it's time for bed—but not before checking the notifications on his phone. He puts his phone next to his bed, abruptly turns off the lights, and proceeds to lie wide awake, tossing and turning until midnight.

To be fair, I suspect that for most of you health-conscious readers, Joe's life might be a bit of an exaggeration. However, in the general population it probably *isn't*.

In fact, here are some shocking statistics of our

current chronic disease landscape which can, in large part, be explained by many of the lifestyle factors exhibited by Mr. Joe:

- Six in ten adults, and 54.1% of children[6], in the U.S. have at least one chronic disease; 40% of adults have two or more[7].

- 42.4% of U.S. adults are obese[8] and 88% of people are metabolically unhealthy[9].

- 34.2% of American adults have metabolic syndrome—a conglomerate of health conditions including, *"elevated waist circumference, elevated triglycerides, reduced high-density lipoprotein cholesterol, high blood pressure, and elevated fasting blood glucose,"*[10]. This condition is associated with increased risk of cardiovascular disease, arthritis, chronic kidney disease, schizophrenia, all-cause mortality, several types of cancer, immunosuppression, and more.

- From 1999 to 2004, *27 million* Americans had an autoimmune condition. Most recent estimates, from 2011 to 2012, show *41 million Americans* have an autoimmune condition[11]. It is reasonable to believe these numbers have followed an upward trend.

- 95% of all COVID-19 deaths had at least one comorbidity, most of which are *lifestyle-related. Within that 95%, the average number of comorbidities was 4*[12]*!* This means that the vast majority of people who died with COVID-19 had an average of 4 chronic diseases.

What does this all mean? While I don't think the solution is as simple as living like the Hadza and forgetting about modern medicine, it's clear that they must be doing *something* right.

Now the question remains: how have we gone from near-perfect metabolic, cardiovascular, and immune health—making 8+ hour hunts in Africa just another day at the office—to multiple chronic health conditions, making 8+ hours of sitting, fast food-eating, and social media-scrolling exhausting? And more importantly, how can we modern humans get the best of both worlds by simulating our evolutionary past in our modern environment to reap the best from both worlds?

Hopefully, you're starting to rid yourself of the black-and-white thinking which plagues the world of health, even amongst well-educated researchers and health professionals. We're human. We tend to make decisions with emotion and justify them with logic. I won't pretend to be free of this bias, but hopefully, I'm aware enough that I can minimize it as much as possible. Now, let's dive into what I refer to as "*the science*".

CHAPTER 2: BEING WARY OF "THE SCIENCE" AND FINDING A HELPFUL ADJUNCT

"It is the mark of an educated mind to entertain a thought without accepting it."
- Anonymous

When I began writing this book, I got into an argument because I didn't think offering free junk food in exchange for a vaccine was a good incentive. From donuts to cheeseburgers, major fast-food chains suddenly felt like they had an important role to play in public health. What a joke. *"But it's a good way to get people vaccinated—it's the most important public health measure right now,"* my objector announced. While I didn't outright disagree with him, I knew there was something off about it—I just didn't know how to articulate it until now. Those incentives were wrong, not because vaccines aren't important, but rather because of the message they sent: by accepting free, hyper-palatable, nutrient-depleted food in exchange for the vaccine, you would stop the pandemic. While vaccines are important, this does nothing but show that some politicians and health officials don't believe anything else matters but vaccinating. As you'll learn in the rest of this book, that's scientifically the furthest thing from the truth. In fact, I'll soon share compelling evidence that poor dietary and lifestyle habits lead to not only more severe COVID-19, but also a *decreased immune response from vaccination.*

Needless to say, as the pandemic has unfolded, many other fallacies and logic-less contradictions have run rampant. Another important example comes from the phrases: "*Listen to the Science*", "*I believe in the Science*", or my favorite: "*Science is real*". That last one just makes me cringe. These phrases have been used extensively by politicians, average Joes, and even some health professionals. On the surface, these declarations sound not only innocuous, but also like honorable and helpful slogans, rather than the virtue-signaling, patronizing statements they often are. The truth is, when most people utter these words, they mean something totally different.

When people say, "*Listen to the Science*", they really mean "*Listen to the cherry-picked opinions of a select few experts which are featured on the nightly news, are readily available to me, and confirm the biases I already had long before the pandemic.*"

When people say, "*Listen to the Science*", they really mean "*Listen to the inherently flawed scientific research often ridden with conflicts of interests, poor methodology, and inconclusive results which I do not understand.*"

If you don't believe this is a real issue, read on. A poll conducted by Franklin Templeton-Gallup, called the Economics of Recovery Study, asked Americans of different political affiliations this question: *"What are the chances that someone with COVID-19 will be hospitalized?"*

Every group, regardless of partisanship, wildly overestimated hospitalization rates, with 28% of Republicans and 35% of Independents believing that *at least half* of COVID-positive individuals must be hospitalized. Strikingly, over *40% of Democrats* believed the rate of COVID-19 hospitalizations to be at least 50%[13]. In other words, Republicans and independents tended to more accurately guess the *true* hospitalization rate: 1 to 5%. What interests me the most about these results is that left-leaning individuals overwhelmingly used the *"I believe in the Science"* slogan. While many may have believed that their opinions and feelings were backed by *"the science"*, the data clearly do not support that. Compared to the hospitalization *estimate*, the *true* hospitalization rate was over *10 times lower*. Don't get me wrong, this isn't an example to bash Democrats and praise Republicans and independents—everyone was off by miles. It merely helps to show that emotions, politics, and media reporting have an *insanely* powerful influence over our perceptions, regardless of the *real* science. Specifically, this survey shows us that the fear-based media narrative that was lodged down our throats was sensationalized, to say the least. I understand the need for alarm at the beginning of the pandemic. However, this same fear-based messaging persisted far too long, probably because it was an easy and relevant way to get our attentions. You might be thinking: *"What's the big deal? It's just a misunderstanding."* The big deal is that most of us perceived this virus to be wildly more dangerous than it was. This false appraisal of risk shaped our emotional states, our political views, our social interactions, and our financial situations.

Although the intention behind "*I believe in the Science*" is indeed honorable, many of the people spouting this slogan do not understand that science is not a rigid ideology, set in stone and never to be questioned. On the contrary, real science is honest, unbiased, and *ever-changing*. One of the core principles of science is to question *everything*.

But our *perception* of science isn't the only thing that's problematic—scientific research itself requires a critical eye. In the search for what is true, systemic flaws created by inherently flawed humans inevitably arise. The reality is, scientific research can be flawed, more imprecise than you think, and inconclusive. The disease model of our modern healthcare system illustrates this fact perfectly, with a single-minded focus on pharmaceuticals and a lack of emphasis on lifestyle. This isn't because lifestyle and dietary interventions don't work. Part of the reason for the lack of focus on lifestyle is the obscene amount of funding to study pharmaceuticals, while less funding goes towards the study of free, non-patentable lifestyle interventions. In fact, the Congressional Budget Office found, "*In 2019, the pharmaceutical industry spent $83 billion on R&D. Adjusted for inflation, that amount is about 10 times what the industry spent per year in the 1980s,*"[14]. How is it that the pharmaceutical business is booming while the chronic disease epidemic has skyrocketed? Don't get me wrong, after interviewing dozens of doctors and health professionals, I believe pharmaceuticals have an important place in medicine––but clearly, they are doing little, if anything, to prevent or reverse chronic disease. I digress.

In this chapter, I'll explain the problems with

scientific research as well as past and present examples of where *"the science"* has been flat out wrong. Without further ado, here's why saying *"I believe in the science"* is the least scientific thing you can say.

The Problems with Modern Scientific Research

Science is awesome, but scientific research can *suck*. By no means am I saying that most scientists are intentionally malicious or that all scientific research is tainted by corruption—that's nonsense. What I am saying is that there are some major problems with the way scientific research is done. So, instead of treating science as a religion—which has been common practice throughout this pandemic—we should acknowledge that there are limitations.

As the U.S. continues to pump out PhD graduates like nobody's business, there simply is *not enough funding*. Though funding, specifically from the National Institute of Health (NIH) increased in the 20th Century, it has since stalled and decreased in the 21st Century[15]. Despite this, young researchers are *entering the workforce* at a faster rate than veteran scientists are *retiring*[16]. If one is fortunate enough to receive a grant, he or she is under pressure to *produce results* to secure future funding[17].

Now, let's look at a couple of papers authored by Dr. John Ioannidis, a Stanford professor of Medicine, Epidemiology, Statistics, and Biomedical Data Science. Dr. Ioannidis published a shocking 2005 paper titled "Why most published research findings are false". Ioannidis states, *"Simulations show that for most study designs and settings, it is more likely for a research claim to be false than true,"*[18]. Due to the methodology, small sample size, and many other factors discussed in the paper, Ioannidis concludes that most findings are not likely to be true. More recently, Dr. Ioannidis published a chilling paper titled "Hundreds of thousands of zombie randomised trials circulate among us." What is a *"Zombie Trial"* you might ask? In his own words they are, *"randomised controlled trials (RCT) that appear to be false and those where the data lack credibility so blatantly that they can be called 'zombies'*,"[19]. Randomized Controlled Trials (RCTs) are near the top of the credibility hierarchy in the sciences since they can tell you if one thing *causes* another. These RCTs can then be compiled into what are called *meta-analyses* to review the totality of evidence. The main takeaway from his paper is that even a meta-analysis of RCTs—which is at *the top* of the hierarchy of evidence—is not free from bias[20]. This makes total sense. If *individual studies* are falsifying or using crappy data, using a *group* of these studies to draw a conclusion will simply yield a giant conglomerate of bias. Ioannidis's paper suggested that hundreds of thousands of these zombie trials exist. The worst part is, this is based on data from only *seven* countries, meaning the real number of zombie trials would likely be *several-fold* higher.

Furthermore, there exists a problem of "wastefulness" in scientific research[21]. What does wastefulness refer to? First, over 50% of papers are *never fully published*, despite findings being relevant and significant[22]. This leaves a vast amount of scientific knowledge in the dark, as researchers may move on to *"more exciting"* and lucrative hypotheses and treatments. Needless to say, the priorities of researchers and patients are often *misaligned*. While the research priorities of patients are *non-drug* treatments, researchers mostly seek to evaluate drugs[23]. What does this actually mean? At each stage of scientific research there is waste, in the sense that many studies are either irrelevant, redundant, biased, or unusable. These findings led this study to conclude that ~85% of investment in research is wasted.

What about conflicts of interest (COIs)? A systematic review paper published in the *British Medical Journal* unsurprisingly showed that, *"Research sponsored by the drug industry was more likely to produce results favouring the product made by the company sponsoring the research than studies funded by other sources,"*[24]. On average, industry-funded drug research tended to exaggerate the efficacy of a drug by 34%[25]. In addition to exaggerating the efficacy of a drug, this conflict of interest-ridden research also tended to *downplay the toxicity* of a drug.

What about the reproducibility of published results? If all of the landmark scientific findings are sound and never to be questioned, shouldn't they be replicable? In other words, can the results of a published study, used to implement dietary guidelines, or determine the safety of medicine, be reproduced in subsequent studies? Unfortunately, the field of psychology and several others are facing a major reproducibility crisis[26]. Why? As one paper puts it, the culture of scientific research breeds, *"(a) incentives for engaging in questionable research practices, (b) a single-minded focus on programmatic research, (c) intellectual hyperspecialization, (d) disincentives for conducting direct replications, (e) stifling of creativity and intellectual risk taking, (f) researchers promising more than they can deliver, and (g) diminished time for thinking deeply,"*[27]. Some researchers and editors of high-profile journals take it a step further. Rather than assuming a study is reliable until proven fraudulent, they propose that we should do the *complete opposite.* These academics propose that biomedical research should be *assumed fraudulent* until proven otherwise[28].

If you think I'm exaggerating, let me bring up a few examples where "*the science*" has been flat out *wrong*.

Big Tobacco: Did We Really Forget so Soon?

I won't spend too much time covering a topic as well known as the tobacco story. As I look around today to see people blindly accepting biased, "science-based" news articles, it seems that we've forgotten the scientific corruption which surrounded tobacco just a few decades ago, which clearly showed the strong grip industry has over scientific research, media, and even government.

If we ever needed a reminder of this fact, it's during this pandemic. In short, this is how the tobacco industry got its way for so long[29]:

- Pregnant women were encouraged to smoke
- Doctors promoted cigarette use
- Addictive nature of tobacco was denied
- Cancer-causing effects of tobacco were denied
- Positive and glamorous marketing was used to attract customers
- Scientific evidence against tobacco products was undermined, twisted, and distorted
- Scientific uncertainty was strategically created to blow smoke (get it?) at public health efforts

Glyphosate: A Controversial Chemical in Our Food, Air, and Water

Monsanto scientists created Roundup in the 1970s to solve the problem of pest control and weed control. You probably have some of it lying around in your garage. Numerous papers have come out since the 1970s, linking glyphosate, and other compounds found in Roundup, to gut permeability and dysbiosis[30], immunosuppression[31], behavioral disorders[32] and neuropsychological[33] disorders, and different types of cancers[34]. Monsanto, an agricultural business giant now owned by Bayer, had done its best to dismiss the detrimental health effects of glyphosate. Using similar strategies as the tobacco industry, Monsanto pulled out all the stops. From ghostwriting scientific papers, to hiding conflicts of interest and beyond[35], Monsanto successfully delayed the inevitable storm of lawsuits—until 2015. In 2015, the International Agency for Research on Cancer (IARC) declared glyphosate as a Group 2A carcinogen, meaning it is: *"probably carcinogenic to humans"*[36].

Glyphosate has been found to adversely affect the gut microbiome[37, 38, 39, 40]. Why is that important? The gut contains trillions of microbes—more than we have cells in our bodies! In short, the gut microbiome is involved with our mood, immune health, metabolism, and essentially *all* aspects of health[41]. What's the issue with glyphosate? This chemical basically works as a sort of selective antibiotic, killing certain microorganisms in our gut which are *fundamental* to health. The worst part is, glyphosate is now being sprayed *directly on food right after harvest* as a desiccant (drying agent), meaning a nice, fresh helping of toxicity alongside your conventional morning oats. Yum.

If you've done a quick Google search, you might have actually found that the U.S.'s Environmental Protection Agency (EPA) claims that glyphosate is *unlikely to be a human carcinogen[42]*. So how in the world did the World Health Organization's International Agency for Research on Cancer (IARC) find the exact opposite?

Fortunately, a paper titled "How did the US EPA and IARC reach diametrically opposed conclusions on the genotoxicity of glyphosate-based herbicides?" sheds some light on this question. The authors write, "*the EPA (1) largely ignored epidemiological studies, some of which reported elevated, statistically significant odds ratios among cohorts that were relatively more highly exposed to GBHs and, (2) placed little or no weight on multiple in vivo GBH genotoxicity assays that reported DNA damage and/or oxidative stress in laboratory animals and exposed human cohorts,*"[43]. Basically, it seems like the EPA ignored some data which showed glyphosate was toxic. For example, in their review, the EPA did not include AMPA (aminomethylphosphonic acid) which is a product of glyphosate (AMPA is a metabolite of glyphosate, meaning that the body breaks down glyphosate into AMPA). AMPA has been shown to cause cellular damage and may lead to increased rates of preterm births[44]. IARC, on the other hand, *did* include the effects of AMPA. In addition, the EPA only focused on 52 *genotoxicity* (ability to damage DNA) studies to make its decision, whereas IARC based its decision on 118 genotoxicity studies. Basically, the EPA's assessment of glyphosate seemed to favor studies which showed no adverse effects from glyphosate and ignore studies which showed negative effects—essentially a form of professional cherry-picking. It's important to note that many of the studies analyzed by IARC had higher levels of pesticide/herbicide exposure than the studies analyzed by the EPA. In other words, IARC and the EPA had different definitions of "real-world" exposure to glyphosate. The EPA argues that the general population is exposed to relatively low levels of glyphosate, while IARC seems to argue that the general population is exposed to relatively higher levels of glyphosate. This also explains the wildly different conclusions. I'll dive deeper into the glyphosate controversy in the chapter on nutrition and gut health.

Butter is Bad, Says Ancel Keys

Let's talk about fat and cholesterol, two heavily vilified components of food—until recently.

The story begins with a man named Ancel Keys. One day, he had a grand idea: cholesterol is *bad*. In the 1950s and 60s, he set out to prove just that. His claim to fame was a research study inappropriately named the Seven Countries Study[45]. Why was this title misleading? Well, the study actually included *more than 20 countries!* When Keys recognized that the majority of countries he surveyed *did not* support his hypothesis, he simply excluded them from the results!

Here are some of the tactics Keys used to get his way:

- Failed to highlight data from the "Seven" Countries Study which did not support his hypothesis
- Claimed he used natural cholesterol and saturated fat (from butter, eggs, etc.) in his experiments, when he actually used *hydrogenated vegetable oils* for several of his studies[46]
- Intentionally did not publish results from the Minnesota Coronary Experiment (MCE), which showed that polyunsaturated fats (from

31

vegetable/seed oils) were just as harmful, if not *more harmful*, than even trans fats[47]! The MCE did show that vegetable oils lowered cholesterol, but *showed no evidence of a decrease in atherosclerosis, death, heart attack, or stroke when substituting animal fats for vegetable oils.* As I'll explain in subsequent chapters, there's some nuance to consider with respect to the health effects of different fats and oils.

Later, the Sugar Research Foundation (SRF), a lobbying group for the sugar industry, aimed to protect the profitability of the sugar industry. How would they accomplish such an *honorable* task? Put the blame solely on cholesterol and fat. In 1965, they sponsored a literature review in the prestigious *New England Journal of Medicine* which put a target on fat and cholesterol, while downplaying the role of sugar in heart disease[48].

Researchers and doctors have dedicated entire books to the *root causes* of heart disease, so I know no matter how I explain this it'll be a gross oversimplification. From my understanding, the reason cholesterol is seen as the cause of heart disease is partly because... well, it is. Ok, cholesterol *is involved* in heart disease. Picture a long tube—this is one of your arteries. Chronic stress, high blood sugar, chronically elevated insulin, hypertension, dyslipidemia, obesity, and other inflammatory conditions can damage the inner lining of your arteries and blood vessels[49]. Sensing an injury, cholesterol rushes in as a *band-aid*. However, if inflammation becomes chronic, more cholesterol lodges on the inner lining of an artery, which leads immune cells (macrophages) to the site of the injury. This process of atherosclerosis (hardening of the arteries) can then lead to heart disease. So, in most cases, cholesterol is supposed to be the *hero*. *We are the ones unknowingly killing ourselves with inflammatory lifestyles.* Of course, there are also genetic components and individual variability with respect to fat and cholesterol metabolism and heart disease, but in general, these mechanisms I described hold true. In fact, several researchers believe that the strongest risk factor for heart disease is the presence of *insulin resistance*, not cholesterol in the blood[50]. Contrary to popular belief, cholesterol which we consume *from the diet* (egg yolks, meat, fish, etc.) can have *very little effect* on the amount of cholesterol in our blood[51]. Our body, like a thermostat, can turn down the amount of cholesterol we produce in response to dietary cholesterol, keeping levels relatively stable. In addition, there seems to be emerging research which shows that *specific types* of cholesterol, such as small, oxidized LDL, may be more responsible for heart disease than others[52]. I'm not suggesting cholesterol is harmless, but rather that the degree to which cholesterol is dangerous seems to be context dependent.

What about saturated fats? Top researchers, scientists, and nutrition experts came together in February 2020 in a workshop titled "Saturated Fat and Health: A Nutrient or Food Approach?" They worked to independently review the evidence regarding the effects of saturated fat on health, as well as the dietary limits on saturated fat set by the United States Department of Agriculture (USDA). This workshop was funded by the Nutrition Coalition, a non-profit organization. The scientists' consensus regarding saturated fat?

"...*there is no evidence that current population-wide arbitrary upper limits on commonly consumed saturated fats in the U.S. will prevent CVD or reduce mortality,"* [53].

In other words, this group of scientists found that the data do not support limiting consumption of saturated fat. To be clear, I'm not saying that *I* know *the truth* regarding saturated fat and cholesterol. I definitely don't carry a stick of butter in my pocket wherever I go. It's important to realize that there is often less consensus than we think, especially among scientists. Therefore, while it's important to be skeptical, it's equally as important to be open-minded, even with topics we think fall under "settled science".

Electromagnetic Fields

Before you bring out the tin-foil hat for me to wear, just know that there are *thousands* of studies which show clear biological effects from Electromagnetic Fields (EMFs). People like to throw around the word *thousands* because it sounds authoritative, and most people won't actually check. In this case, there are *truly thousands* of studies which show that even extremely low frequency EMFs and radiofrequency radiation—like cellphones, cell towers, and WiFi routers—have a biological effect on our bodies. For decades, the physicists liked to say, *"These gadgets can't possibly damage humans—they don't have enough energy to break DNA."* In the chapter on EMFs, you'll see why this erroneous assumption has come to bite us in the butt in recent years.

Kale is Good… No Wait, it's Bad

If you look hard enough, you can find studies which stand in direct opposition to each other. One paper concludes red meat is cancerous, while another concludes the *carnitine* in red meat is a powerful antioxidant[54]. One paper may tout the vegan diet as a cure-all, while another points out that vegans have higher nutritional deficiencies and developmental issues[55]. One paper calls Kale a superfood[56] while another shows that large amounts of raw kale contribute to goiter[57], an enlargement of your thyroid gland. A paper may conclude that dietary saturated fat causes heart disease, while another concludes that the consumption of saturated fat actually leads to lower all-cause mortality (more on that later).

You can always find at least one study, doctor, or scientist which will uphold your biases. Believe all animal products are bad? There exists a legion of vegan doctors, citing studies which tell you exactly what you want to hear. Believe keto is the optimal diet for humans? There exists an equal and opposite tribe of expert keto doctors waiting with a pile of hand-picked studies to confirm what you think you know. This is known as cherry-picking, and it happens on all sides of virtually any argument. As long as there is open debate, this human tendency isn't all that problematic. Another way to get around so much bias is to look at meta-analyses and reviews—basically, studies of many studies. This is important when reviewing what's (probably) most true. The problem is, as I explained earlier, that sometimes even meta-analyses cannot be trusted.

Unfortunately, there are political, social, and economic forces at play which make it difficult for scientific research to actually be *real science*. The political force should be what stands out to you the most, as it seems to be the most prevalent force getting in the way of science nowadays. Over one hundred years ago, we were asking for the separation of church and state.

Now, we should call for a separation of science and state. When science and politics do mix, science should influence politics, but *never* the other way around as it has throughout this pandemic.

***

Supplementing Science with Sense

If we (sometimes) can't even trust the top of the evidence hierarchy in science—meta-analyses of randomized controlled trials—now what?

We should totally dismiss science. The end...

I'm totally kidding.

Instead, we should raise an eyebrow (or two) to any claim that we hear which is backed by "*the science*". We should use common sense, (reasonable) personal experimentation, and our evolutionary past as adjuncts. For example, I saw a tweet the other day from a dermatologist who said something along the lines of: "*There is no safe amount of sun exposure*". Ooh. Scary. But wait a second, if our early ancestors have been constantly exposed to sunlight since the dawn of time, does that mean all of them were walking, talking tumors? Did we all suffer from melanoma before the invention of modern sunscreen? Or is this dermatologist just repeating what he's been told, emotionally attaching to a belief, and ignoring our evolutionary history?

If this example holds true, then humans must have *barely* survived up until today. In other words, until modern science came along, our poor ancestors knew nothing about the world and were always on the brink of death, disease, and starvation. Right? Wrong.

How is it that ancient Indian medicine (Ayurveda), thousands of years ago, understood fasting to be a powerful therapy for numerous ailments[58]?

How did ancient populations know to soak, sprout, and ferment foods to enhance nutrient availability and neutralize plant defenses? How did ancient medical systems know meditation to be a powerful modulator of mental, physical, and immune health? How did ancient philosophies understand that we are "energetic" beings (now widely accepted, but referred to as electromagnetic)? How did early practitioners of Traditional Chinese Medicine know tea to have anti-inflammatory, cognitive-boosting properties? In ancient writings, tea was referred to as "cold", having the ability to lower "fire"[59]. While the word inflammation was not around back then, it was somehow understood that chemical constituents found in tea (catechins, polyphenols, etc.) had powerful anti-inflammatory properties which could stave off diseases. And how did early hunter-gatherer populations understand the concept of "like supports like"? Now known as *homostimulation*, this concept is defined as the process by which eating organ meats will support the corresponding organ in our bodies. There is now emerging scientific evidence in support of this idea. Beef heart, for example, contains CoQ10, an essential cofactor for a healthy heart[60].

So, how did they acquire so much wisdom without a *single* peer-reviewed, randomized, double-blind, placebo-controlled study? Before scientists could perform statistical gymnastics to determine whether something was significant, our ancestors relied on thousands of years of common sense, personal experimentation, and wisdom. I want to be clear that I'm not saying we shouldn't do science. On the contrary, these ancient realizations arose from thousands of years of *genuine curiosity* and *honest observation*—in other words, *real science*.

***

After my critique of scientific research, something about this book probably doesn't seem quite right. I reference several hundred scientific papers in this book, many of them meta-analyses and reviews. I just told you the plethora of problems in the sciences, so why should you trust what I'm saying? The short answer: *you shouldn't*. As a human being, much like yourself, I am not free of biases either. The purpose of this book is to question—to show that there is rarely such a thing as "settled science". While I'm grateful for science, I'm not convinced we'll find the ultimate truth about health in a textbook. Instead, I've come to believe in the power of personal experimentation. Rather than a one-size-fits-all approach to health, people should be encouraged to change up their diet and lifestyle in response to tracking *their own* biomarkers (cholesterol, DNA, CRP, blood sugar, etc.). I believe this *is the future*.

At this point, it should be clear that I didn't write this chapter to throw as much crap on science and modern medicine as I could wrap my hands around. Instead, I hope to reverse the path we seem to be currently on: one of blind acceptance and close-minded scientific dogma with a religion-like fervor. That's *not* science, that's *"The Science"*.

CHAPTER 3: FIRST, DO NO HARM (?)

Before I get to the meat of this chapter, I need to tell you something I really didn't want to admit: I began this book totally enamored by the "back to nature" movement. Let me explain why that's relevant. Rather than using the amazing supercomputer located above my shoulders, I let my biases overpower my capacity for deep, rational thinking. Before writing this book, I had a deep distrust in modern medicine *as a whole*, and therefore, I came to a simplistic conclusion in my head: *"All modern medicine is bad"*. As I look back, I now ask myself: how could I *not* believe this? If the previous chapter taught you anything, it's *fool me once shame on you, fool me twice shame on me*. Much of biomedical research, and the drugs which result from it, are guilty of our skepticism. However, at the time, I didn't realize just how devoid of black-or-white the world was—everything is complicated and deserves context. The same goes for modern medicine. So, when I took the decision to write this book, I made a promise to myself: I will commit myself to being level-headed and *honest* with myself and with you.

This commitment was especially important when it came to investigating a topic as apparently murky as the COVID-19 vaccines. Therefore, if you're polarized on the pro-vax side, don't worry—this chapter won't be another anti-vax rant. If you're polarized on the anti-vax side, don't worry—this won't be another pro-vax rant either. Instead, I'm going to do something much less flashy—simply give you as much information about the COVID-19 vaccines as possible. A few disclaimers first: I will never be able to do this section justice, because, as I explained earlier, science is always evolving and therefore, this section cannot stay evergreen. In fact, as time goes on, this section will probably become *irrelevant*—but that's ok. Instead of merely spewing information about the vaccines, I hope to show you how I went about challenging my biases—from as many angles as possible—in my objective search for the truth. Additionally, by the time you read this, it is very likely that my opinion will have evolved along with new scientific knowledge. Yours should too.

Let's say you identify as "pro-vax." You might feel hatred, resentment, and even disgust towards the "anti-vaxers". Let's say you identify as "anti-vax". You probably feel the same feelings against the other side. But it's important to realize a few things. There are *many* people—dare I say, *most* people—on both sides who can't argue with logic why they so rabidly believe in their stance.

It's clear that anyone who has brought up *any* concern (rational or not) about these new vaccines has been almost immediately condemned as an *anti-vaxer*. That word carries so much negative charge that it totally discredits the person, even though they could indeed have a logical, scientific concern. This boggles my mind. Instead of discussing *what* the person is saying, the *"anti-vax"* label—when it is wrongly used––dismisses the person as a pseudoscientific, tin foil hat-wearing conspiracy theorist. The worst part is, this has increasingly been happening to health professionals with legitimate concerns. While I doubt that there is any useful way to use the words *anti-vax* or *pro-vax*, if you were to use it properly it should be for people who, *no matter the amount of evidence*, will not change their opinion. If a vaccine fails, injures many people, and does not reduce severity of a disease, those who do not acknowledge this could be correctly labelled as "pro-vaxers". On the other hand, if there is a vaccine which dramatically reduces the spread, severity, and is safe across a wide age range, people who dismiss the vaccine's efficacy and safety could be correctly labelled as "anti-vax". For better or worse, I now understand that humans are emotionally driven. We might think we're being unbiased, but as soon as a label is incorrectly placed on someone—and it most likely *is* incorrect—we shut down our brain centers for rational thought and dismiss people as wackos. What a waste of human potential.

Though it will always be a learning process, I have found a few simple ways to navigate this, and many other controversial topics, with people I do not agree with. Instead of trying to *beat* someone in an argument to show off my intellectual and verbal prowess, I have learned to take a breath and remind myself that we probably both want the same thing: *the truth*. And when you find that your actions don't reflect that commitment, ask yourself why that is. Not only does this relieve pressure and promote a healthy debate, but it also makes for a much less combative and hostile environment. I also ask myself an important question to put myself in their shoes. For example, why would someone who is labelled as "*anti-vax*" think that vaccines are dangerous? Were one of their children disabled from a vaccine injury? Did they witness a loved one have a stroke shortly after vaccination? People should not be dismissed, ridiculed, or gaslit for their painful experiences as they have been throughout this pandemic, unless your goal is to further polarize people.

***

At the beginning of the pandemic, I often heard the following argument in support of the COVID-19 vaccines: "*Vaccines have been proven to be safe. We've used them for decades and they are one of medicine's greatest achievements,*". Depending on which side you're on, you might have a different visceral reaction to those sentences. The problem with this argument is that, while it may hold true for vaccines in the past, it did very little to inform us about the novel mRNA vaccine in question—at least, at the beginning of its development. Assuming that a novel drug or therapy is safe without extensive testing is the opposite of the Precautionary Principle in medicine, which states, "*…one should not act when there is no scientific proof that no harms will result from a medical act or a policy decision,*"[61]. Now, I understand that medicine must act quickly in unprecedented times. However, at the very least, *both sides* of the story should have been *discussed*—the benefits *and* risks. In other words, as soon as the vaccine was available, we should not have put the cart before the horse. Nonetheless, politicians were quick to discuss mandates when we didn't even fully understand the possible mid- to long-term side effects, natural immunity, or SARS-CoV-2 itself.

I found this phenomenon to be true as I went into my doctor's office to do my annual check-up. When I asked about the COVID-19 vaccines, I received zero information on the risk/benefit ratio of the vaccines *for me*. Instead, I was met with a blind, near-idolatrous faith about how wonderful the COVID-19 vaccines were—a few weeks after they became available.

Here's why I found that somewhat troubling. Several doctors have mentioned that, as students, they were told that 50% of what they're taught in medical school will be wrong after they graduate—they just won't know which 50%. Due to this phenomenon, Dr. Dave Sackett, the "Father of Evidence-Based Medicine", adds that, "...*the most important thing to learn is how to learn on your own,*"[62]. The problem is that it can be difficult for many conventional doctors to stay up to date on the latest research when they have so much paperwork, have many patients to see, and their practice is centered on—as one of my podcast guests put it—giving a "pill for the ill". In fact, a 2017 study showed that the average physician spends over 6 hours of his/her day split between office visits, administrative tasks, phone calls, and writing prescriptions[63]. The problem? It's estimated that around 7,287 clinically-relevant studies are published each month. This would take an estimated *600 hours per month* to review[64]!

But how the heck does this relate to vaccines? When my doctor never mentioned *any* concerns he had about the vaccines, it unfortunately wasn't because evidence didn't exist that the *unknown risks* could outweigh the possible benefits for my age, health status, and whether I was previously infected. This doctor simply wasn't well-informed or was willfully ignorant, hiding behind a fanatic belief in "*The Science*" rather than critically assessing scientific research on a *case-by-case basis*. In fact, at the time of writing this book, the Joint Committee on Vaccination and Immunization—an independent expert committee which advises the United Kingdom—has stated that they do not advise healthy people 18 years of age and younger to get the COVID-19 vaccine[65]. Several other countries have followed suit.

Because you've likely dealt with the same one-sided experience—whether it be for, or against the vaccines—this is my effort to bring you information which you might not have heard, whether you have decided to get vaccinated or not.

Short Term vs. Long Term

In the short term, the vaccine appears to be safe for most people. In the long term, the short answer is: *who knows?* This is not a hyperbole—even the experts can't possibly answer that question! There's no data! Though most side effects seem to happen in the first few weeks to months after vaccination with previous vaccines, this is a new pharmaceutical. For many people, especially elderly, immunocompromised, or those with comorbidities, the vaccine benefit seems to far outweigh the risk. However, everything deserves some context, which is why one-size-fits-all recommendations are short-sighted and potentially damaging—just look at the food pyramid[66].

The first scientific concern I came across when I began to investigate is a phenomenon known as

Antibody-dependent enhancement (ADE) of disease[67]. ADE can occur when vaccination makes a person more likely to have severe disease when he or she comes in contact with the actual virus. How does that happen?

A dive into the literature on ADE revealed that there are neutralizing antibodies and non-neutralizing/binding/enhancing/facilitating antibodies (they couldn't even agree on one name). Think of a balance, with neutralizing antibodies on one side and enhancing antibodies on the other. When the scales tip toward enhancing antibodies, ADE is more likely to happen, since these antibodies can actually *facilitate* uptake of a virus into a cell. In other words, these types of antibodies can make it easier for a virus to infiltrate cells. Therefore, a vaccine which leads to abnormally high levels of enhancing antibodies can lead to ADE.

A paper published early in the pandemic in the *International Journal of Clinical Practice* explains, "*Vaccines for SARS, MERS and RSV have never been approved, and the data generated in the development and testing of these vaccines suggest a serious mechanistic concern: that **vaccines designed empirically using the traditional approach** (consisting of the unmodified or minimally modified coronavirus viral spike to elicit neutralizing antibodies), be they composed of protein, viral vector, DNA or RNA and irrespective of delivery method, **may worsen COVID-19 disease via antibody-dependent enhancement (ADE),*"[68]. This was a rational concern *at the time*, which unfortunately, my doctor did not mention.

A subsequent paper sought to address the possibility of ADE with the Delta variant, which had not been specifically evaluated. Researchers explained

45

that, for the original Wuhan strain, the balance was tipped in favor of *neutralizing* antibodies in vaccinated individuals, meaning the vaccines tended to be effective, safe, and rarely caused ADE. However, the research team found that neutralizing antibodies have a lower affinity for the spike protein in the Delta variant, while *enhancing* antibodies have a higher affinity[69]. This means that the "good", neutralizing antibodies which neutralize a virus cannot do their job properly, while the "bad", enhancing antibodies which make disease worse, are better able to stick on to the Delta strain. They argued that this could potentially make a vaccinated individual more likely to get sick, more transmissible, or more prone to severe disease.

ADE has not been thoroughly evaluated with newer strains of SARS-CoV-2*.

Though often used interchangeably, SARS-CoV-2 refers to the virus, whereas COVID-19 refers to the disease caused by SARS-CoV-2.

Trans-Generational Effects

Another concern I came across has to do with the potential for trans-generational effects, which means that we may not see the effects in the people who get the shot, but we *may* in the children of those who get the shot.

A paper published in *The International Journal of Molecular Medicine* explained:

"Of note, the question remains whether humanity is currently willing to pass on potential devastating diseases to future generations due to the present need for the speedy development of a vaccine, bypassing adequate long-term and transgenerational safety testing," [70].

What's missing in that paper is that the virus

itself may also cause transgenerational effects. No one can know for sure whether these effects will occur or not but it's important to be aware that it is a possibility. Everyone must be as informed as possible and decide (with their own physician) which risk they are willing to take.

Is Natural Immunity Not a Thing Anymore?

I've been amazed with the dismissal of natural immunity, despite evidence that natural immunity is protective. Schools, employers, and businesses which require vaccination have totally dismissed immunity obtained through infection. Even though natural immunity can be heterogeneous (not everyone gets the same protection after infection), so can immunity conferred through vaccination. More well-known examples of this are seen in the elderly, immunocompromised, and obese. In other words, those who are *disproportionately vulnerable* to this disease, show significantly *less* of an immune response to vaccination[71].

What I'm about to say is not suggesting you go out and try to get infected but bear with me. A preprint study discussed, "*...natural immunity confers **longer lasting and stronger protection against infection, symptomatic disease and hospitalization** caused by the Delta variant of SARS-CoV-2, compared to the BNT162b2 two-dose vaccine-induced immunity*," [72]. This same study showed that one was *13 times* more likely to be reinfected and *27 times* more likely to develop symptoms in the never-infected, *fully vaccinated* group than if one had previously been infected. Furthermore, never-infected, vaccinated individuals were also much more likely to be hospitalized than those who were

47

naturally infected and unvaccinated. In other words, if you recovered from COVID-19, you were—on average—much less likely than vaccinated individuals (who hadn't been infected) to be hospitalized.

Furthermore, a paper published in the journal of *Clinical Infectious Diseases* studied the risks of vaccinated vs unvaccinated Health Care Workers (HWCs). They found, *"Compared to unvaccinated seronegative HCWs who had the highest rates of infection, incidence was 98% lower in unvaccinated seropositive HCWs (adjusted IRR [aIRR] 0.02 [95% confidence interval {CI} < .01–.18; P < .001]), and 67% lower following a first dose in previously seronegative HCWs (aIRR = 0.33 [95% CI .21– .52; P < .001]), with no symptomatic infections seen following a second dose (Figure 2). Incidence was also 93% lower in vaccinated previously seropositive,"* [73]. In other words, unvaccinated Health Care Workers (HCWs) who had antibodies to SARS-CoV-2 got infected at a similar rate to fully vaccinated individuals. In addition, people who had been vaccinated *and* infected had the highest levels of antibodies. Since governments and many businesses are now simply requiring vaccines (without checking if someone was previously infected), it makes zero sense to dismiss natural immunity, as the protection from each are similar.

But the natural immunity story doesn't end at just antibodies. In fact, T cells, immune cells which help create long term immunity to disease, have been found at least 6-9 months after a SARS-CoV-2 infection[74]. Another paper, published in the journal *Cellular & Molecular Immunology* found that, *"...natural induction of SARS-CoV-2 adaptive immunity confers a robust protective effect for **at least 1 year**, similar to what has also been reported in infections by other related coronaviruses,"* [75]. A study published in the journal *Nature* showed that T-cells were formed even in the absence of a detectable viral infection. The researchers explain, *"Data now suggest that the majority of infected individuals develop robust and **long-lasting T cell immunity**, which has implications for the durability of immunity and future vaccine approaches"*[76]. Therefore, most of those who have been exposed to SARS-CoV2 seem to have robust, lasting immunity. Even mild cases seem to develop immune memory against SARS-CoV-2[77]. When comparing vaccine efficacy to protection conferred by natural immunity, natural immunity provides an **80-95%** protection from reinfection—similar to the vaccines[78].

Finally, from a mechanistic standpoint, natural immunity may have an advantage. Unlike the mRNA vaccines which only target the *spike protein*, our body recognizes several other parts of the virus, making it a more "comprehensive" record of the virus. What do I mean by that? It's now well understood that SARS-CoV-2 encodes the following proteins: the spike protein, nucleocapsid, membrane, and envelope protein[79]. If the mRNA vaccines only "train" the immune system to recognize *one* component of the virus (the spike protein), it makes sense that newer strains of the virus may "learn" to evade vaccine-induced immunity. The theory is that, in general, natural infection will lead to broader immunity than vaccines as a result. A study which analyzed immunity 8 months after infection stated: *"The immune response to natural infection is likely to provide some degree of protective immunity even against SARS-CoV-2 variants… Thus, vaccine induction of CD8+ T cells to **more conserved antigens such as the nucleocapsid, rather than just to SARS-CoV-2 spike antigens, may add benefit to more rapid containment of infection as SARS-CoV-2 variants overtake the prevailing*** *strains*,"[80]. Allowing the body to recognize more than just the spike protein may lead to greater protection to variants.

So… why are we ignoring natural immunity?? The short answer is: a mix of incompetence, bias, and political and economic forces which are beyond my current understanding.

After so much talk about vaccines and natural infection, an important question inevitably arises: have we reached herd immunity? Well, according to the vaccine mandate cult, the only way to reach herd immunity is through vaccination. The number of people with immunity required to reach herd immunity seems to be anywhere from 60-85%, depending on who you ask. A major study published in *The Journal of the American Medical Association* collected 1,594,363 blood samples from all 50 states in order to determine how many people had been infected and carried antibodies to SARS-CoV-2. The research group found that combing vaccine-induced immunity with natural immunity yielded about 83% population immunity[81]. Some scientists, however, believe herd immunity, regardless of vaccination, is impossible due to new variants which are vaccine-resistant, lack of evidence regarding vaccines preventing transmission, and several other reasons[82].

Again, this isn't suggesting you go out and get infected—depending on your health status, your risk could vary. Instead, I'm saying that our natural immunity to COVID-19 is relevant, more powerful than once believed, and should stop being dismissed. If one has been infected, getting a COVID-19 vaccine afterwards may be an unnecessary risk, especially for low-risk, young, and healthy individuals who have antibodies and/or T cells to SARS-CoV-2. Immunity, regardless of how it is obtained, seems to be *the* truly important metric.

Transmission

The vaccine trials have not directly shown reduced transmission, which is a common argument for mandating vaccinations. In fact, scientists admit, "*…what has been poorly studied in the phase 3 pre-registration studies and in the post-authorization clinical trials, is whether the vaccinated subject infects with the same frequency and probability as an unvaccinated subject,*" [83].

In addition, a real-world study titled "Shedding of Infectious SARS-CoV-2 Despite Vaccination" showed that viral load—the amount of virus that can be found in your body—is similar in both vaccinated and unvaccinated individuals. Importantly, they also note: "***Vaccinated and unvaccinated persons should get tested*** *when symptomatic or after close contact with someone with suspected or confirmed COVID-19*"[84]. Colleges and businesses, *take note*—follow the actual science. I digress.

Why is viral load important? Infected individuals with more viral load are thought to spread the virus to more people[85]. Another study conducted by University of Oxford scientists stated, "*Peak viral load therefore now appears similar in infected vaccinated and unvaccinated individuals, with potential implications for onward transmission risk,*"[86]. Furthermore, Brown and colleagues found that the cycle threshold (Ct) was similar in vaccinated and unvaccinated individuals. Ct refers to the number of cycles needed to detect the virus. The greater the Ct value, the lower viral load in an individual (i.e., the less viral particles someone is carrying around). This is how PCR tests work, meaning that those with similar Ct values should have similar viral load. Therefore, the main purpose of the vaccine is to ideally lower *severity, hospitalizations, and deaths*—NOT transmission. In fact, a CDC study found that 74% of the symptomatic cases in a Massachusetts outbreak were in those who were fully vaccinated[87]. This isn't necessarily reflective of the entire population, but it's important to know that vaccinated individuals can still get and transmit SARS-CoV-2.

Finally, a recent study published in the *European Journal of Epidemiology* found no association between increases in COVID-19 cases and vaccination rates. Specifically, "*The lack of a meaningful association between percentage population fully vaccinated and new COVID-19 cases is further exemplified, for instance, by comparison of Iceland and Portugal. Both countries have over 75% of their population fully vaccinated and have more COVID-19 cases per 1 million people than countries such as Vietnam and South Africa that have around 10% of their population fully vaccinated,*"[88]. In other words, high vaccination rates did not mean lower COVID-19 cases. In fact, they found that *some* countries with the highest vaccination rates have more COVID-19 cases. To be fair, just because case numbers are not significantly different between highly vaccinated countries and those with low vaccination rates does not mean vaccines have not had a positive effect on hospitalizations or deaths. The authors conclude that finding additional pharmacological *and* non-pharmacological approaches to deal with the pandemic is important.

Some researchers speculate that the time until viral clearance is lower in those who are vaccinated, meaning that, on average, vaccinated individuals may be infectious for less time, indirectly lowering the chance that a vaccinated individual will infect others[89]. This has not been directly studied however—especially with regards to new variants. In addition, this question has not been studied comparing those with natural immunity versus those who are fully vaccinated.

So, why are colleges, businesses, and restaurants treating unvaccinated, previously infected individuals as if they have the bubonic plague?

Risk vs. Benefit

As is human nature, we often tend to look at things in the simplest way possible. This human tendency has led many people to believe that risk of getting a severe case of COVID-19 is the same for everyone. However, the risk is *different* for each subgroup of people, whether you are in your 60s, in your 20s, have a certain vitamin D status, are physically fit, or you have comorbidities[90]. After this chapter, I will demonstrate to you that many of these comorbidities have a profound impact on your risk of death from COVID-19 and are *strongly* influenced by lifestyle habits.

The infection fatality ratio—the proportion of deaths among all those infected with a disease—is, indeed, different for every age group, as estimated by the CDC[91]: 0.002% (0-17 yrs), 0.05% (18–49 yrs), 0.6% (50–64 yrs), 9% (65+ years)[92].

In addition, a meta-analysis published in the *European Journal of Epidemiology* showed that an American aged 0-34 is *3.75 times more likely to die from a car accident than dying after getting infected with SARS-CoV-2*[93]. If you've been following the news, you've likely heard that soundbite and dismissed it as a wild exaggeration. The data show that this is no exaggeration. The most shocking part is that this is *only* considering *age* and not any of the immune-supporting habits I'll share in the rest of this book. Other countries studied seem to have similar infection fatality rates as well, such as Spain, Portugal, and Norway[94]. The age-specific estimates of infection fatality rates are also very similar in a paper published in the journal *Nature,* titled "Age-specific mortality and immunity patterns of SARS-CoV-2"[95].

Death, however, is *not* the only important metric. While risk of death may be low in certain populations, long term side effects may still be prevalent and can interfere with everyday activities. These symptoms, collectively known as long COVID-19, include, brain fog, hair-loss, headache, fatigue, attention disorder, and many more[96]. The vaccines have shown efficacy in lessening the risk of developing these effects. Although there are currently no studies––and they may not ever exist––on lifestyle habits and risk of long COVID-19, it is reasonable to believe this risk would also greatly decrease with proper lifestyle and dietary habits.

95% Vaccine Efficacy?

In writing this book, I came across a website called www.thennt.com. NNT stands for the Number Needed to Treat. In other words, this organization of independent physicians and researchers seeks to ask a simple overarching question: How effective are pharmaceutical drugs in treating patients? The research compiled by this organization was a great starting point for me to delve into the research myself.

Again, with respect to the Pfizer vaccine, it

seems to be safe in the short term. The research suggested that it was not clear in the trial studies how many were tested and confirmed for COVID-19 because the documents do not describe how many people were tested in the control and vaccine group[97, 98]. What does this mean? Worst case, this means that the efficacy is lower than reported. Regardless, the NNT team still recommends vaccination at the time of writing this book.

There's also an important distinction to be made between absolute and relative risk reduction. Most of the vaccines available at this point have a *relative* risk reduction (RRR) of ~95%. Sounds pretty amazing right? However, what many vaccine-mandate zealots miss is that the *absolute* risk reduction (ARR) is around 0.84%[99]. In other words, the Pfizer vaccine prevents *one* infection for every 119 people vaccinated. The authors of a paper published in the journal *The Lancet* clarify, "*Although the RRR considers only participants who could benefit from the vaccine, the absolute risk reduction (ARR), which is the difference between attack rates with and without a vaccine, considers the whole population. **ARRs tend to be ignored because they give a much less impressive effect size than RRRs: 1.3% for the AstraZeneca–Oxford, 1.2% for the Moderna–NIH, 1.2% for the J&J, 0.93% for the Gamaleya, and 0.84% for the Pfizer–BioNTech vaccines,*"* [100]. From my understanding, this apparent statistical manipulation *isn't* cheating, as many anti-vaccination zealots have suggested. Both the RRR and ARR tell us something different, and neither one should be ignored. For a detailed breakdown on this subject, I highly recommend looking into Dr. Mobeen Syed's medical lectures on this topic.

I'll end the section on vaccines with an interesting quote from a study published in the *International Journal of Molecular Medicine*:

"*The main target population for a vaccine is the most vulnerable demographically: the elderly with high comorbidities and dysfunctional immune systems. Yet, the test demographic population being used for the initial clinical trials is the relatively young and healthy population (as discussed below). This leads to uncertainty regarding the efficacy of the trial, raising issues as to how the results from a young healthy population can be extrapolated to an elderly and vulnerable population. Additionally, in myriad cultures, it is the elderly who sacrifice for the benefit of the young. This tradition is being inverted in the present accelerated testing regimen,*"[101].

Stop Using Horse Dewormer (?)

No, Ivermectin is not just a horse dewormer, like many media outlets, governments, and politicians have claimed. I despise half-truths—especially from supposedly credible institutions to which we give our trust. Scientists won the Nobel Prize in 2015 for discovering that ivermectin safely and effectively worked *in humans* against tropical diseases[102]. So, why have doctors been ridiculed and cancelled because of their stories about using ivermectin to treat COVID-19 patients successfully? For starters, there were some misguided individuals who actually used veterinary-grade ivermectin, and NOT human-grade ivermectin! Also, there were no clinical trials which specifically showed ivermectin's efficacy and safety for COVID-19 treatment. Skepticism is great, but as the data have rolled in, scientific skepticism has turned into willful blindness and myopia. I have seen firsthand ivermectin help people lessen the severity of COVID-19 as well as get people out of Long COVID. I understand this is anecdotal, but data now exist in the form of controlled trials.

Ivermectin is an affordable, safe, and *generic* drug. The past few decades of research have revealed antiviral and anti-inflammatory properties of ivermectin as well[103]. The interesting thing about ivermectin is that it is *generic*. Instead of a brand-name medication which is expensive and is owned by one company, generic drugs are cheap and widely available. In other words, there's not a lot of money to be made from ivermectin.

However, I'm not suggesting ivermectin is the panacea, like many others have claimed. While several meta-analyses and reviews seem to show very promising results, others seem to be total letdowns. For instance, one study based on 18 randomized controlled trials suggest: *"...large, statistically significant reductions in mortality, time to clinical recovery, and time to viral clearance. Furthermore, results from numerous controlled prophylaxis trials report significantly reduced risks of contracting COVID-19 with the regular use of ivermectin,"* [104]. Another study based on 24 randomized controlled trials showed, *"reduced COVID-19 infection by an average 86%,"* [105]. In addition, a systematic review of ivermectin showcases its relative safety, antiviral, and anti-inflammatory mechanisms—published all the way back in June 2020[106]. On the other hand, one systematic review and meta-analysis which used 10 randomized controlled trials found that ivermectin did not significantly improve outcomes in COVID-19 patients with mild symptoms and thus should not be used[107]. In addition, many of the positive outcomes with ivermectin used a shotgun approach, administering ivermectin, vitamin C, vitamin D, quercetin, zinc, and a bunch of other compounds. Therefore, it's hard to say which compound is responsible for the positive effects.

Of course, as a single person I truly can't know the entirety of the evidence regarding ivermectin. But I do know enough to say that the scientific conversations surrounding ivermectin should NEVER have been censored, nor should scientists discussing ivermectin have been ridiculed. There is no logic behind doing so. Almost everyone wants the same thing—to help save lives and get people healthier. In the search of what will accomplish such a goal, we cannot afford to silence *anyone*. Although you might end up rightfully censoring a couple of crazy cranks every now and then, you will also censor *good, honest* scientists who have cutting-edge information to share, which could be potentially *lifesaving*.

I've come to realize that there are almost always two sides to every story. Ivermectin seems to be no different.

Final Concerns and Thoughts

Several articles published in the *British Medical Journal* (BMJ) do a great job of explaining many of the concerns with the methodology of vaccination trials and data reporting bias[108]. In addition, these articles[109] point out that the vaccine trials are studying the wrong endpoints—specifically they raise the fact that the trials were not designed to show whether the vaccines save lives, prevent infections, or prevent transmission[110]. In addition, a paper published in the prestigious journal *The Lancet,* titled "COVID-19 vaccine efficacy and effectiveness—the elephant (not) in the room," also explained that phase 3 Pfizer vaccine trials only tested the ability to prevent mild or moderate COVID-19 infections, NOT hospitalizations and deaths. Therefore, the numbers from these trials are not based on the vaccine's ability to prevent death, hospitalization, or transmission, but rather *a mild case.* In fact, a study published in the *New England Journal of Medicine*, one of the most prestigious medical journals, showed results 6 months out from being vaccinated with Pfizer: "*During the blinded, placebo-controlled period, 15 participants in the BNT162b2 group and 14 in the placebo group died*". In other words, in this gold standard study, vaccine deaths were not significantly different from deaths in unvaccinated individuals. Other data out of Israel, however, do seem to suggest that the vaccine *is* effective in reducing severe COVID-19, hospitalizations, and death[111]. Again, my point with this chapter and book is not to discourage someone from getting vaccinated. Instead, I would like to curb the arrogance with which people declare that there is only *one* solution to the pandemic and that any dissidents are insane. The science is not settled.

At the time of writing this book, the vaccines in the U.S.—except for Pfizer which was recently approved—are currently under Emergency Use Authorization and will likely not finish their safety trials until May 2023[112], meaning true *informed consent* about the vaccines is literally impossible. Informed consent means you are aware of all of the benefits as well as possible risks. No one knows these risks yet because the mid- to long-term data simply do not exist. In addition, there is NO formal control group to assess long term effects of these vaccines. What does this mean? Basically, the gold standard of scientific research (blinded placebo-controlled trials), is not being used for these vaccines any longer. This is because several weeks after the vaccines were approved for emergency use, most participants in the control group were offered—and received—the vaccines. Long story short, now we may not know the mid to long term effects of these vaccines in a formal study because the control group is no longer a true control group.

Next, vaccine companies also have immunity from legal action if one has a severe adverse reaction to the vaccines. The Congressional Research Service states that, "...*the Public Readiness and Emergency Preparedness Act (PREP Act) authorizes the Secretary of Health and Human Services (HHS) to limit legal liability for losses relating to the administration of medical countermeasures such as diagnostics, treatments, and vaccines,*" [113]. Basically, if you have a severe side effect to the vaccines, there's no one to blame. You cannot sue the pharmaceutical companies which injured you because the government has provided them protection. However, I would not be quick to jump to the conclusion that this protection is nefarious.

Finally, the CDC decided to stop tracking breakthrough cases (cases in vaccinated people). Why they chose to do so is somewhat nebulous, but many experts warn that not tracking the cases of vaccinated individuals does not make sense if the goal is to get ahead of the virus.

Needless to say, all of the previous sections are—or were at one point—scientifically valid concerns with the vaccines. You might think to yourself: "*Well, why haven't I heard many scientists talking about this? No way our public health officials just overlooked this, but some 20-year-old college kid somehow didn't.*" The answer is something you probably already know: the news doesn't do a great job of covering current events in an unbiased manner. The truth is, many scientists, doctors and PhDs did share these same concerns about the vaccines. In my experience, the people who do not work in healthcare and are not fully informed were more likely to believe vaccines should be mandated for everyone. Trust me, I understand that this idea is well-intentioned. However, a deeper dive into the nuances of mandating a new vaccine makes this idea questionable at best, and authoritarian at worst (at least, at this moment in time). Why? For starters, mandating a new vaccine (and creating punishments for those who don't) could backfire, especially for those of lower socioeconomic status. Punishing people who have not yet been vaccinated (in places where vaccines may also not be widely available) widens the gap of inequity. Mandating these new vaccines without enough data could also fuel anti-vaccine sentiment. If someone just *tells* you what you *must* do (and holds your livelihood hostage), without properly explaining why, how likely are you to do it? Mandating the vaccines may not even make sense given the fact that natural immunity is relevant and likely as powerful as vaccination.

Much to my surprise, many of the doctors and nurses I've personally spoken to, as well as the scientists whose research I have read—no matter their political views—*do not* support mandating this new vaccine, even if they have supported previous vaccines or are fully vaccinated themselves. Please open your mind up to the fact that you *can* have someone who supports vaccination but is also *against* mandating these new vaccines.

Now, I want you to take a guess at the most vaccine hesitant group in the United States... You might imagine a crazy conspiracy theorist, uneducated person, or a rabid, pickup truck-driving Trump supporter—as many media outlets would have you believe. While this stereotype may also be true, researchers from Carnegie Mellon University and the University of Pittsburgh surveyed 5 million U.S. citizens across different demographics to find out which groups were most COVID-19 vaccine-hesitant. They found that the group with the highest vaccine hesitancy was highly educated people with PhDs[114]. In fact, there's an organization known as the Coalition Advocating for Adequately Licensed Medicines (CAALM) which petitioned to the FDA to *not* approve the COVID-19 vaccines until extensive safety testing is completed. CAALM is made up of medical doctors, PhDs, and editors of major scientific journals. Regardless of this petition, and others like it, the Pfizer vaccine has been approved.

***

It should be clear that the previous sections are not arguments that the vaccines do not work. Although vaccine efficacy has dropped significantly with alpha and delta variants, especially for Pfizer, this doesn't mean that they are useless[115]. A 60-year-old with type 2 diabetes and high blood pressure would likely be a no-brainer for being vaccinated. An 18-year-old with no health conditions and has been previously infected? Maybe not.

I've spoken to people on both extremes of the vaccine debate. The common theme is one of hatred, mockery, and disgust against "the other side". I can understand that feeling. People want to blame *someone* for all that we have gone through this past year. I'd like to refer people on all sides playing the blame game to this saying: *When you point a finger, there are three more pointing back at you.* The truth is, it's highly nuanced and complex. Even researchers and doctors admit that they do not have the answer to end the pandemic—they know it would be incredibly arrogant to say so. Vaccinating everyone is, of course, a possible solution but it may not be the only, or the most reasonable, way out.

As you can see, it's not only the tinfoil hat-wearing "conspiracy crazies" that question vaccine efficacy and safety. Many of the studies I referenced come from prestigious journals like *Nature, The Lancet,* and the *British Medical Journal.* We have reached a point where simply dismissing more doctors as quacks because they have expert opinions outside of the mainstream narrative is becoming *absurd.* I think it seems controversial to have concerns about this vaccine because we often see the extremes on the news—a radical *"pro-vaxer"* or a fanatic *"anti-vaxer".* How exciting is it to see rational, calm debate about the pros and cons of a therapy or drug? Not so exciting, is it? This choice is personal and should be discussed with a competent physician who understands the data, risks, and benefits well. Sadly, there seem to be few allopathic physicians I've personally come across who understand most of what I've written in this book.

At the end of the day, here is what has served me the most—listen to *everyone,* as no *one* person has the whole truth. BUT be *really careful* to not get carried away by people who speak in absolutes, do not add context to their claims, speak in black-and-white terms, and make blanket statements. Don't expect any one person to give you *"The Truth"* with a capital "T", but rather pieces of the truth. Learn to challenge all ideas you hear in order to extract what's really true from as many experts as possible. And the next time you hear someone say *"Listen to the experts"* or *"Listen to the science"* just know they're not referring to the totality of science, but rather their own biases under the guise of science.

Without further ado, let's dive into all of the modern lifestyle factors which have crippled our health, leaving us vulnerable to many chronic diseases, as well as COVID-19.

RESOURCES

1. Physicians for Informed Consent
2. Dr. Marty Makary
3. For COVID-19 Protocols created by doctors visit the Front Line COVID-19 Critical Care Alliance (FLCCC) and BIRD Group
4. Dr. Pierre Kory
5. Dr. Paul Marik
6. Dr. Roger Sehuelt
7. Dr. Geert Vanden Bossche
8. Dr. Peter Doshi
9. Dr. Zubin Damania
10. Dr. Bret Weinstein
11. Dr. Suneel Dhand
12. Dr. Peter McCullough
13. Dr. Mobeen Syed

CHAPTER 4: IMMUNE HEALTH BEGINS IN THE MIND

It's no secret that stress plagues our modern world. An average 9 to 5 job basically *guarantees* you a steady amount of psychological stress throughout the day. We're constantly bombarded by notifications, expectations, emergencies, and stressful news headlines. The current state of the world has simply added fuel to the flame.

If you have been watching any sort of news lately, you know what I'm referring to. Most news headlines read something like this: *New Coronavirus Strain,* or *It's not Over: The Second Wave,* or *Case Numbers Skyrocket,* and my favorite: *Why You Should Worry about COVID-19.* Meanwhile, alternative media articles have gotten bashed for headlines such as *The Importance of Vitamin D in COVID-19 Prevention and Treatment,* or *How Micronutrients Support Immune Health,* and *What you can do to Decrease Risk of Severe COVID.* Spot the major differences? While I don't fully condone the latter (some of those alternative health articles are totally full of it), they at least serve an important purpose: they don't contribute to the worldwide *nocebo* effect initiated and perpetuated by most media outlets. You've probably heard of a *placebo* effect: a phenomenon which occurs when people who don't receive a treatment/drug still get better because they *believe* they will get better. Well, a *nocebo* effect is the opposite: when a person gets sicker because of a belief that he/she will get worse.

The point is, bad news have gotten views, while good news have gotten either censored or labeled as dangerous. Again, I don't believe everything that has gotten censored has been because *"the powers that be are suppressing information!"*. Nah. I think some of the claims made by people who went viral weren't actually evidence-based, but I still don't think they should have been censored. That's a slippery slope. Science is advanced *only* by open discussion. Remove expert opinions and you eliminate problem-solving potential. There were legitimate opinions that were diametrically opposite to the media narrative of fear, fear, and more fear. At the beginning of the pandemic, it's understandable—we don't know what we're dealing with. But this same sensationalized news reporting continued well past the point of being reasonable. Dr. Knut Wittkowski, biostatistician and epidemiologist with 20+ years of experience, Dr. Zach Bush, triple-board certified physician, Dr. Bret Weinstein, evolutionary biologist, Dr. Peter Doshi, editor of the BMJ, and countless other health professionals have gotten censored for their expert opinions. The Social Media Overlords of Absolute Truth deemed *expert opinions* as "medical misinformation" simply because these viewpoints about the pandemic differed from

"The Science".

So, where does that leave the average non-scientific citizen getting bombarded with sensationalized news headlines? In a state of perpetual fear and stress. Let's talk about what these emotions are in a biological sense. Fear is a *stress response*, meaning it activates the sympathetic portion of the nervous system which releases stress hormones. Our immune systems are sensitive to stress hormones, such as cortisol. While short term stress may *enhance* some parts of the immune system and *impair* others, chronic stress is more clear-cut. When stress is chronic, *global immunosuppression* occurs[116]. To put it simply, when there's a lion chasing you, all energy goes to escaping that immediate threat. Fight-or-flight mode puts the digestive system, parasympathetic nervous system, and the immune system on the backburner. In the modern world, that lion usually takes the form of a demanding boss or parent, screaming children, fear-laden news headlines, or negative thoughts.

Why are these emotions such a bad thing in the long term? Chronic anxiety, fear, and stress have been shown to:

- Reduce white blood cell activation, increase lymphocyte death, and reduce B and T cell production[117]
- Down-regulate genes involved with immune response and contribute to *thymus involution[118]*. The hub of T-cell regulation, the thymus is an often-forgotten organ. Involution refers to atrophy of the thymus, leading to wimpy T-cell production, which leaves the immune system impaired
- Increase risk of depression, cardiovascular

disease, autoimmune disease, and upper respiratory infections as well as increase inflammatory immune response[119]

In fact, the *second strongest lifestyle risk factor* for dying with COVID-19 was the presence of depression, PTSD, anxiety, obsessive compulsive disorder, or other neuropsychiatric conditions[120]. You read that right. Right after *obesity*, people with anxiety and fear-related disorders were much more likely to die with COVID-19.

Basically, *chronic stress is bad news* if you want a robust and healthy immune system. The good news is——contrary to the mainstream news headlines—there is *a lot* you can do about it.

Identify Stressors

First, what I'd recommend is simply this: *identify* stressors, *determine* what you can do about them, and *identify* what is in your control. Write them down, talk about them—but whatever you do, resist the urge to ignore them. Then, think about what you can do about them. Are they directly in your control or are they in your environment? You may not be able to control the state of the world but think about what is in your control. There's a lot more than you think. You *can* improve your health starting today. You *can* further your skills and expertise in any field you want. You *can* choose to develop new habits. Hopefully, this book will help you with several of those. Also remember that this book is just a guide and not a prescription by any means. Seek out help! Find health professionals who will work with you rather than lecture at you. You do not have to go through your health journey alone.

Breathe—Outside!

We can live for days without food and water, but we can only live for minutes without air. Not surprisingly, breathing is one of the foundations of human life and health. Despite its absence from our conscious minds most of our lives, it is an important proxy for health. Next time you're in a stressful situation, check your breathing. Is it shallow? Is there a longer inhale than exhale? Do you feel out of breath? Interestingly, the breath follows from our emotional state, but it can also be reverse engineered. What do I mean by that?

If you are stressed out and you find yourself shallow breathing, focus on breathing deeply through your nose and you'll find that your emotional state will follow the calm, relaxed breath. When I feel stressed, anxious, or angry, I have found it helpful to focus on the breath. Doing so brings me back into self-awareness, allows me to reassess my state of being, and—most importantly—allows me to *change* my emotional state. My favorite breathing techniques are as follows:

- *Bhastrika followed by Rechaka.* These breathing techniques come from a practice called *Pranayama* used in yoga. *Bhastrika* is done by sitting upright and cross legged on a mat or bed, forcefully inhaling through the nostrils, and simply letting go of the breath when exhaling. Find the rhythm that works for you––experiment with quick breathing and slower breathing. Start by doing 30 consecutive breaths. Do *rechaka* right after, as it is the antithesis to the more stressful *bhastrika*. *Rechaka* activates the parasympathetic (rest and digest) portion of the nervous system. Simply inhale through the nostrils effortlessly and *extend* the exhale as long as you can, lightly pursing your lips. This breathing technique is very similar to the Wim Hof method, though there are some slight differences. I recommend searching for guided video tutorials.

- *4-7-8 breathing.* Inhale for 4 seconds, hold for 7, exhale for 8 seconds. This is great for reducing anxiety and stress.
- *Box breathing.* Breath in for four seconds, hold for four, exhale for four, hold for four, then repeat. Find the number which works best for you. Four seconds is merely a suggestion.

In addition to the mental benefits, nitric oxide (NO) is released, which improves blood flow, can lower blood pressure, and is antiviral[121]. Make sure to breathe through your nose and not through the mouth to allow more NO to be released[122].

While these breathing techniques will undoubtedly bring benefits, doing them outdoors brings a much more enhanced experience. While indoors you likely have some amount of dust, maybe some mold, built up air pollution, and definitely some toxic cleaning products, the outdoors has its own air fresheners—plants.

In addition, there's another compelling reason to spend time in nature. A Japanese practice known as *Shinrinyoku,* or forest bathing—basically, spending some time in nature—has unsurprisingly been shown to have remarkable effects on human health. Several studies have found increased activity of natural killer cells—our body's defense against tumors and virus-infected cells—as well as enhanced sleep as a result of spending time in nature[123]. Many researchers believe this is partially due to the presence of *phytoncides*, chemicals which are excreted by trees and plants which exert powerful effects on our immune systems[124]. Several of these studies were in people who spent days immersed in nature, so if you can go camping—go for it. If all you can do is take a hike every once in a while, do it. Just spend time in nature. Check out my podcast episode with Dr. Bartlett Hackenmiller to learn more.

Finally, as a selectively impatient person who wants to see results instantly, it pains me to tell you the following: it may take more time than you think for breathwork to exert its effects. You can think of it as a sort of medicine—if the dose is too low, it just won't work. If you're feeling stressed out but only take two minutes to breathe, you might not see any noticeable effect. Give yourself at least 5 to 10 minutes daily, especially if you're having a rough day.

Meditate

I like to think of using our minds like lifting a weight. When you lift a weight, you're contracting a muscle. Some contraction is good, as it allows for stimulation and breakdown of the muscle—the first steps in building muscle. However, if it is *constantly* contracted, there can be NO repair, and therefore, no growth. Now, compare that to the constantly busy minds of the 21st century.

Our minds are in a state of pretty much constant contraction (i.e., stress). What is the antidote? That's where meditation comes in.

Here is how you get started
- Start cross-legged on a mat or carpet. Bonus points if you meditate outdoors.

71

- Take a few deep breaths
- Start from the top of your head and scan all the way down your body, releasing any tension. Bring conscious awareness to sensations, such as heartbeat, digestion, and breathing—but *don't try too hard!* This is a critical piece of the exercise—refraining from trying too hard.
- Acknowledge thoughts and feelings but let them pass through your awareness. When you realize you're lost in your problems rather than simply *being* without expectations, acknowledge them, feel the feeling, and let it go. Again, no forcing is required. Simply allow thoughts and emotions to come and go. View them from a third-person perspective without judgement. Practice makes *progress*. Don't expect to reach enlightenment in the first 3 minutes of meditating.

An important note: Be consistent. I cannot express that enough. Even 5 minutes a day will be beneficial, as long as you are consistent. Set a goal for 31 days, 21 days, or even just 7 days. Here is the most crucial information regarding meditation: once you feel it start to slowly work, *do not stop*. I have made that mistake countless times. I've consistently meditated for a few weeks and *slowly* start to feel better. Then, I suddenly decide it's not important enough to take 5-10 minutes out of my day. *That* is when the benefits stop. Consistency is key with meditation.

But where's the evidence, you might ask? As

you've probably guessed by now, I don't have a mental block against an idea which hasn't been peer-reviewed or double-blinded in a study. For thousands of years, meditation has been a part of many cultures. In addition, my own personal experience always takes precedent over, or at least complements, the existing research. Luckily, ample data do exist on the health benefits of meditation. The following results come from a review on mindfulness meditation which included 20 randomized controlled trials with more than 1600 participants[125]. Here's what the researchers found:

- **Decreased *Nf-kB* transcriptional activity**. *Nf-kB* regulates pro-inflammatory genes. Lower activity means less of these genes are expressed which may lead to *lower inflammation*.
- **Decreased CRP levels**. C-Reactive Protein (CRP) is a common biomarker used to measure inflammation in the body. Lower CRP corresponds to lower inflammation.
- **Increased Telomerase activity**. Telomerase is an enzyme which helps maintain the integrity of telomeres—the caps on the ends of chromosomes (picture the ends of shoelaces). Why is that important? As chromosomes replicate, the telomeres wear down—which is why telomere length is associated with aging. A positive association exists between telomere length and longevity. However, in recent years, telomeres have become less relevant in predicting longevity, as better methods have been developed.
- **Down-regulated HPA axis**. The hypothalamic-pituitary-adrenal (HPA) axis is

responsible for the activation of the stress response and maintaining proper levels of glucocorticoids (such as cortisol, the well-known stress hormone). Dysregulation of the HPA axis occurs in times of chronic stress, anxiety, and panic disorders. Meditation has been shown to have a "calming" effect on the HPA axis, leading to balanced levels of stress hormones.

Light Makes you High?

In addition to all the other directly immune-supporting benefits of sunlight which I'll discuss in the next chapters, there's also an interesting *anti-stress* component to simply lying in the sun. Soaking up the sun releases *beta-endorphins*—our bodies' naturally-produced opioids[126]. Similar to the molecules which create a runner's high, *beta-endorphins* create a natural feeling of relaxation.

In addition, I make sure to get outside in the sun as soon as I wake up, or at least look at very bright light. This is an important cue to your body that it's time to be awake, release certain hormones, and inhibit others. We're built to run on a 24-hour circadian cycle. Light is one of the crucial cues to our eyes and skin during the day, which sets your body up for the proper release of hormones throughout the day. This simple habit also leads to better sleep.

Food

Omega-3 fats have been shown time and time again to be *anti-inflammatory, anxiolytic,* and *anti-depressive*[127]. I'd recommend getting them from food, since many fish oil supplements are iffy at best. Here are the top ways I consume omega-3:

- Wild-caught salmon
- Wild-caught sardines, anchovies, and mackerel
- Hemp seeds
- Soaked flax
- Soaked chia seeds
- Walnuts

I usually stick to small fish like sardines, since they have the lowest amount of heavy metals *and* the highest omega 3 content. Staying away from chia and flax seeds might be a good idea if one has digestive issues. Fiber and other plant compounds—contrary to popular belief—can actually cause bloating, constipation and other uncomfortable digestive issues[128]. Be aware of how *you* respond to certain foods. *Bioindividuality* is the name of the game. Though many plant-based advocates claim that you can get enough omega 3s on a plant-based diet, it's not exactly true. There are three different types of omega-3 fats: ALA, EPA, and DHA. Plant foods are typically good sources of ALA, whereas animal foods are rich sources of DHA and EPA, both of which are important for brain health[129]. ALA *can* be converted into EPA and DHA, *but* it's estimated that only around 5% of ALA converts to EPA and DHA[130]. However, if you're dead set on being vegan, you *can* get DHA and EPA from algae. But for most people it's probably more practical to eat some sardines and salmon.

Next, let's talk about sugar. Most people know reducing sugar consumption and replacing it with whole foods, may be the simplest, yet most effective ways to improve metabolic health. However, they may be unaware of the link between highly refined carbohydrate consumption and mental health. Some research has shown similar brain activation in substance abuse, demonstrating loss of impulse control and increase of stress-driven eating when eating refined carbohydrates[131]. Otherwise stated, if you're used to eating refined carbs, how hard is it to eat just *one* bite of a doughnut? In addition, poor blood sugar control––when your blood sugar looks like a rollercoaster—is associated with anxiety-like behaviors[132].

Magnesium

As you read this book, you'll probably see magnesium mentioned in almost *every single chapter*—for good reason. Around 20% of the U.S. population has a magnesium deficiency, with some estimates as high as 50% of the population[133].

Some of the contributors to this epidemic are processed food consumption, chronic stress, and the quality of the soil.

First, processing food strips it not only of magnesium, but also fiber, valuable minerals, and vitamins. It's estimated that about 80% of magnesium is lost during food processing[134]. That's why you see refined flours fortified with synthetic vitamins and minerals.

Next, magnesium has an interesting relationship to stress. Magnesium has been shown to have anti-stress effects. In fact, there seems to be an *inverse* relationship between stress and magnesium status[135]. The more stress one has, the less magnesium is present. The directionality is not clear, however: does one get stressed and lose magnesium or does a magnesium deficiency lead to a stressed-out person? Either way, magnesium seems to be important for mental health and the stress response.

Finally, in the past few decades, the soil has become depleted of minerals and vitamins, such as iron, magnesium, and vitamin B12, just to name a few. Intensive modern agricultural practices, such as tilling the soil, monocrop agriculture, pesticide use and increase in global CO_2 concentrations are largely to blame. In fact, a 2012 study estimates that the amount of magnesium in North American wheat has decreased by ~27%[136].

Therefore, due to magnesium's absence from the conventional diet, many people may benefit from supplementation.

As with every supplement, diet, or lifestyle change, the response is based on the individual. Check with your physician to see how something like magnesium could interact with a medication or health condition. If you want to find out more about specific forms of magnesium, check out my two-part podcast series on magnesium.

Reduce Coffee Consumption (?)

First, there's the issue of mycotoxins. These compounds are formed by mold and are present in many coffee brands. While some sources say mycotoxins are not found in significant amounts— since we can filter them out through our liver—we need to take a step back and analyze that claim. Unless you live in a pristine grassland untouched by industry, mycotoxins are NOT the only toxin in your life. Alcohol, pesticides, herbicides, toxic chemicals in water, shampoo, and more, *all* get filtered through the liver. Therefore, while mycotoxins may not be, in themselves, that problematic, they just *might* be in a real-world setting. In fact, toxicologists know that both *acute, high dose*, as well as *chronic, low dose* exposure to toxins can be problematic[137]. If you're like most people and you will drink coffee until the day you die, I'd look into buying an organic brand. The next tier would be finding a coffee brand which is third-party tested for pesticides, mycotoxins, and other contaminants.

Next, coffee is a diuretic, basically meaning it makes you pee more. Why is that relevant? This means that every cup of coffee you guzzle depletes you of essential minerals (including magnesium and sodium). Unsurprisingly, caffeine may result in subjective experience of jitteriness and anxiety. How does that play into mental health and immune function? Caffeine increases the amount of cortisol (stress hormone) and adrenaline (involved in fight/flight response) in the body[138]. Therefore, heavy coffee drinking (5+cups a day) may be a detriment to both mental and immune health over time.

However, there are associations between moderate coffee consumption and increased longevity[139], reduced oxidative stress, reduced risk of cardiovascular disease, type 2 diabetes, and liver disease[140]. So, observe how your body and mind reacts and decide what's best for you.

Vitamin C

As everyone probably knows by now, Vitamin C is important for immune function. Interestingly, it's also an important component of our stress response. The adrenal glands are mainly known for their role in making stress hormones. It turns out, that vitamin C (ascorbic acid) is highly concentrated in the adrenal glands[141]. It has been shown to moderately decrease blood pressure, subjective experience of stressful events, and cortisol, one of the stress hormones[142].

I personally use a whole foods source of vitamin C, such as camu powder or acerola cherry powder and take one dose in the morning and another at night, rather than one mega dose.

Gratitude

Gratitude has to be one of the most overlooked ways to improve health and quality of life across people of any socioeconomic status. Here's what the research shows about gratitude:

- Makes you get better at feeling gratitude (duh)[143]
- Improve subjective sleep quality[144]
- Reduce stress[145]
- Lowered depressed mood, reduced fatigue, and lowered inflammatory markers such as CRP, TNF, and IL-6[146]

Now, it can be strangely difficult to feel *genuine* gratitude at times, especially since we live in an era where we can open up our phones and instantly see people in their garage with their Lamborghini, for instance. Here's one trick I've picked up to really *feel the feeling* of gratitude: first thing in the morning, journal one or two things/people you're grateful for; picture them clearly in your mind; now, imagine what life would be like without them; finally, give thanks again that they are *still* in your life.

Laughing and Loneliness

Mental and spiritual health is often neglected in the world of "biohacking", nutrition, and fitness, but I'd argue it should actually be front and center. This is especially true when it comes to immune health.

Here's one study where participants watched funny cat videos for an hour[147]. Natural Killer (NK) cells are a type of white blood cell which makes up the innate immune system. After watching a funny video, NK cells had *significantly higher* activity. What does that mean? NK cells were better able to do their job, ruthlessly destroying tumor cells and cells infected with a pathogen. The most shocking part was: these effects were still noticeable 12 hours *after* watching videos of cats playing the piano (ok, I actually don't know what videos they watched).

Next, if you've read any popular media article on loneliness, you likely know it's bad news for our health. In most of these articles, loneliness is mainly mentioned as having an *indirect* negative effect on health. In other words, being lonely makes you more likely to do behaviors which are unhealthy, such as eating crappy foods and skipping exercise[148].

While these indirect effects are without a doubt significant and harmful, some argue there are indeed *direct* effects of loneliness. It's no question that humans are social creatures—without our ability to engage with others positively, humans would never have survived ice ages, warring tribes, etc. In fact, social isolation and loneliness are now thought to directly lead to heightened anxiety and depression, increased risk of cancer, cardiovascular disease, and greater susceptibility to infectious diseases[149]. So, make time for friends, phone calls, zoom calls, stand-up comedy, and—if you're into it—funny cat videos.

Emphasize Sleep

It's no surprise that stress causes poor sleep.

Therefore, by following this chapter, sleep should improve. However, in addition to the mental aspects of proper sleep, there are also important physical components which can help you snooze your way to health.

RESOURCES
1. Dr. Gabor Mate
2. Dr. Joe Dispenza
3. Dr. Jordan Peterson
4. Sadghuru
5. Smiling Mind app
6. Headspace app
7. Ten Percent Happier app
8. Wim Hof Method
9. Holotropic breathing
10. Dr. Mark Atkinson
11. Waking Up app by Sam Harris
12. SOMA Breath by Niraj Naik

CHAPTER 5: SNOOZE YOUR WAY TO HEALTH

Let me take you back to one of my earliest memories. It isn't a wondrous memory of the zoo—when I pressed my face against the dirty window of a chimpanzee enclosure for the first time. It also isn't a sentimental memory about being pushed on the swing by my mom or dad. Instead, the memory I'm referring to is about my crappy sleep. I was, at most, 4 years old. Picture a small bed covered with Spider Man sheets; toys scattered all over the floor, which, unfortunately, was tile. Why was that unfortunate? Many nights, I would often wake up after *rolling off of my bed* onto the cold, hard tile floor—all 35 pounds of me. This was so recurrent that my parents started to put pillows all over the floor! If that weren't enough, my parents would often tell me that I'd speak in my sleep—as I grew older, I would do so in different languages! Clearly, my sleep sucked. Fast forward to my teens and, though I wasn't falling off my bed anymore, my sleep continued to suffer. After eating dinner with my family, I would dread going up to my room for yet another night of trying to tyrannize myself to sleep. When I finally managed to fall asleep, I'd wake up at least 5 times a night. And when I was rudely woken up by my alarm, I simply couldn't get up.

Unfortunately, it's not just me who suffered from terrible sleep. It's estimated that as many as 50%[150] of people worldwide have sleep apnea, insomnia, or other sleep disorders[151]. What's the problem? Chronic sleep deprivation increases the risk of type 2 diabetes[152], cardiovascular disease[153], depression[154], obesity[155], and anxiety—which all *independently* raise the risk of severe COVID-19. Starting to get the picture? Everything is connected to everything else. This is why I, and so many others, rabidly preached about getting healthier at the start of the pandemic. Who knows how many deaths could have been prevented if our top public health authorities had taken the time to emphasize the importance of our lifestyle habits at the start of the pandemic? Actually, scientists *have* come up with an estimate, but you'll have to wait until the end of the book to find out. I digress.

Several review papers have shown the impact of sleep on inflammation. Cytokine storms have gotten major attention this past year, as they seem to be one of the key features of severe COVID-19. Cytokines are inflammatory signaling proteins involved in the immune response. They're essential, but if they get out of hand, collateral damage ensues, leading to systemic inflammation. Indeed, a pro-inflammatory cytokine called Interleukin-6 (IL-6) increases after *several nights of poor sleep,* as does C-reactive Protein (which isn't a cytokine but is a measure of inflammation and correlates with a cytokine storm) [156]. This isn't just a hypothesis anymore. A recent study showed that those with chronic lack of sleep pre-COVID-19 diagnosis, were at an *8.6 times* greater risk of having more severe symptoms than those who got 7 to 8 hours of sleep[157]. A study published in the *British Medical Journal* found that for every additional hour of sleep, the risk of COVID-19 dropped by 12%[158]. Obviously, the return-on-investment levels out—your risk of COVID-19 does not just keep decreasing infinitely as you sleep more and more!

Another study found that those who had quality sleep had improved functioning of T cells—which are necessary for a healthy immune response. T cells have been found to be important in forming a lasting immune response towards SARS-CoV-2[159].

Now, let's get into the good stuff. Here are a few things I do before bed and during the day to tell my body and mind it's time to sleep.

Breathe

In the modern world, it's remarkably easy to get caught up in stress, feeling like there's always more to do, things are not the way they should be, and ultimately that we are not the way we should be. As we get swept up by this current of stress and anxiety, we often unconsciously start shallow breathing. I've sometimes noticed it in myself whenever I'm writing articles, doing work, or reading. Sometimes, I won't even shallow breathe, I'll literally just *stop breathing* completely. And I used to wonder why I often felt stressed out doing homework...

This feeling of the everyday grind often follows you into the bedroom, leaving your mind running at 100mph while you try to tyrannize yourself to fall sleep (which, as I've learned, isn't very effective). My favorite breathwork techniques for sleep are: 4-7-8 breathing (4 sec inhale, 7 sec hold, 8 sec exhale), 10 sec inhale and 10 sec exhale, 4-8 breathing (4 sec inhale, 8 sec exhale), and just simply slow, deep nasal breathing. Refer back to the previous chapter for more breathwork.

Separate Your Work Environment from Your Sleep Environment

I returned to college after more than a year off and found that my sleep had once again returned to… absolute shit. After experiencing incredible sleep months before—which I had missed out on for most of my life—I was beyond frustrated by my inability to fall asleep and stay asleep when I returned to school. Though *many* factors were at play, I realized that one major factor was mental. I had gotten used to doing all of my homework in my room. No wonder I found myself unable to turn off my brain at night. I was associating my room with unreasonable homework assignments and reading that I didn't want to do! I now do most of my work at the library and consciously designate my house as a place for rest and fun. As soon as I walk in, I know it's time to wind down.

A simple but effective tool to make the transition from high stress to relaxation is simply to read. For extra credit points, read something inspirational, such as affirmations. Why? At night your brain waves change from alert and focused, to slow and *suggestible*. After reading a few pages, I often find myself unable to keep the book upright, much less keep my eyes open.

Meditate

A great way to end the day and quiet the chatter of the mind, especially before sleep. Many people who walk to their bed in hopes of having a restful slumber often have a whirlwind of thoughts rattling around in their head. How on Earth do you expect to sleep with worries, fears, and anxiety still shooting through your veins?

That's where meditation can be an incredibly useful tool. Look back at the section on meditation, as well as the resources, in the previous chapter for more.

Block Blue Light

Within your eye, you have photosensitive retinal ganglion cells (a mouthful, I know) that detect blue light and influence your 24-hour circadian rhythm. During the day, sunlight has a naturally higher ratio of blue light compared to other wavelengths of light. This, along with the intensity of the light, signals wakefulness. However, in the evening—due to the angle at which light hits the Earth—the frequencies of light that reach our eyes are more orange-red with very little blue. Just think of a sunset. Unsurprisingly, the modern world gets in the way of our health with alien light. Instead of a calming sunset, we constantly bombard ourselves with bright light from LEDs (which emit a high proportion of blue light). So, it may be 9PM, but by having the lights on, we're essentially telling our body "*Hey, wake up!! It's midday!*"

So, what can you do about the inevitable bombardment of blue light? For starters, you could replace your lightbulbs with dim amber or red light bulbs. That's a good step, but it's not optimal. I recommend wearing long sleeves and pants (skin is light-sensitive as well) and investing in a pair of amber, blue light blocking glasses. I have truly noticed a difference in sleep quality when I throw on my glasses at night. I also notice much less eye strain and fatigue when using my devices, watching TV, or looking at any other screen. Ideally, we would give up all light when sunset came around, but you and I both know that ain't happening. Check out my resources page at livedamnwell.com/resources to look at the glasses I recommend for daytime and nighttime.

Consume the Calm.

Magnesium has been shown to have an anxiolytic effect on the body and the mind[160]. It is necessary for hundreds of biochemical reactions in the body. What does that mean in terms of sleep? To put it simply, magnesium may allow one to reduce feelings of anxiety more easily. This is important because feelings *lead to thoughts* which *lead to feelings* which lead to more thoughts, and so on.

If you know what anxiety—or a negative thought pattern—feels like, you know it can easily become a vicious cycle. Therefore, if you nip it in the bud and give your body a tool to reduce the *feelings* of anxiety, it just makes sense that less negative thoughts may arise, and less anxious feelings will as well. This is especially important at night at a time when the mind can be overactive. I highly recommend you check out my two-part podcast series on all of the different forms of magnesium, dosing, and nutrient interactions.

Bone Broth??

There's a reason why a nice warm broth was given as a medicine for many of our ailments as kids. Not only is it helpful for a cold, but it can also be surprisingly helpful right before bed. Bone broth, especially grass-fed beef bone broth, contains a mighty dosage of glycine, a "calming" amino acid. In fact, this is why I take magnesium glycinate—a magnesium bound to glycine—right before bed. This amino acid––in addition to its ability to increase our master antioxidant glutathione—has been shown to reduce core body temperature and work as an inhibitory neurotransmitter[161, 162]. Your body temperature drops at bedtime anyway, suggesting that glycine could speed up the process. Since inhibitory neurotransmitters, such as GABA,[163] are associated with *lower anxiety and calm*, this leads to even better sleep.

L-Theanine

L-theanine is an amino acid found in green tea. It seems to increase alpha brain waves in individuals with high anxiety[164]. How is that relevant to sleep? Alpha brain waves are typically associated with relaxation, making it a good tool to have before going to bed. L-theanine also seems to moderately improve sleep quality in those with ADHD[165], anxiety, and depression[166]. Finally, 200mg of L-theanine reduced the stress response in individuals exposed to stressful stimuli[167]. L-theanine may not have a super impressive effect on your sleep in isolation. However, when combined with other habits/supplements, L-theanine seem to work synergistically.

In my experience, it can also be great to have after overdoing caffeine. L-theanine seems to reduce the jitteriness and stress which comes from having a little too much of your favorite Starbucks drink.

Stay Cool

As I said before, your body works on a 24-hour circadian rhythm. As I discussed earlier, there's a drop in core body temperature at night. So, turning on a fan, throwing off the blanket, or taking a hot shower before bed can ease you into your body's natural circadian rhythm. *A hot shower if you want to be cold?* Yes, taking a hot shower *vasodilates*, meaning your blood vessels dilate. This process releases heat and cools you down.

Sungazing

Ok, don't actually look directly at the sun. Every morning, go outside and expose as much skin as possible to the sun. This is great for people who have fair, sensitive skin since the morning sun is the least likely to cause a sunburn and is a great way to build up resilience to the sun. Through your skin and eyes, the right formulation of sunlight (colors, brightness, and ultraviolet light intensity) tells your body it is the beginning of the 24h wake/sleep cycle.

But how is that gonna help my sleep? To put it simply, if your body knows it is morning, that will set your body up for the release of hormones at just the *right* times *throughout* the day. Here's how it works. Serotonin—a neurotransmitter associated with regulating mood—is produced in response to sunlight[168]. Since serotonin is the precursor to melatonin (the sleep hormone), getting adequate sun exposure throughout the day can improve sleep. If you cannot get sunlight exposure, at least expose yourself to artificial bright light in the morning to get your circadian rhythm going.

In addition, vitamin D, produced in our skin from sun exposure, has been shown to influence how we sleep. Supplementing vitamin D has not only been shown to improve *sleep quality*, but also reduce sleep latency (the time to fall asleep), and sleep duration[169]. Though scientists are not yet clear as to how vitamin D exerts these effects, Dr. Stasha Gominak, a pioneering neurologist who I had the pleasure of interviewing on my podcast, theorizes that vitamin D interacts with the microbiome and neurotransmitters. Specifically, the theory holds that vitamin D can affect levels of acetylcholine, an inhibitory neurotransmitter in the brain. I recommend checking out my interview with her to learn more.

My Shotgun Recipe For Sleep

If you've noticed, many of the sleep-enhancing supplements or habits I've mentioned aren't the panacea for sleep. In other words, doing just one of the habits in this chapter in isolation probably won't lead to amazing sleep. If you're an avid tea drinker, you've likely seen teas touted for their ability to make you sleepy. If you look closely at these teas, the main ingredient which is to blame for inducing sleepiness is often chamomile tea. But what is it about chamomile tea that causes drowsiness and anti-stress effects? A compound called *apigenin,* or *biapigenin* seems to be the culprit[170]. It seems to reduce anxiety by increasing GABA, one of our main inhibitory neurotransmitters in the brain[171]. Chamomile and apigenin have been shown to significantly improve sleep quality and improve generalized anxiety disorder symptoms[172].

Here's the recipe I use whenever I need to ensure a good night of sleep: in hot water, I steep 2 or 3 teabags of chamomile tea, add honey to taste, and add 200-500mg of L-theanine. If I really desperately need some good sleep, I wash down capsules of 1-4g of glycine and 100-200mg of magnesium L-Threonate along with it. Why the honey? Research has found that a small, high carbohydrate meal one hour before bed significantly decreased sleep onset[173].

If tea isn't your thing, you can always consider supplementing apigenin, along with the other supplements and a spoonful of honey.

Sleep Anxiety

After years of dealing with terrible sleep, it seemed like my research and self-experimentation was paying off. I was finally sleeping like a normal human! But just when I thought I had cracked the code on sleep, it got even worse than before. What happened? It all began when I came across the work of several prominent sleep scientists who shall remain unnamed. These well-meaning sleep advocates truly *catastrophized* getting even *one* rough night of sleep. Reading between the lines, their core message sounded like our lives should revolve entirely around our sleep! If you didn't choose sleep over *all* else, you were setting yourself up for anxiety, high blood sugar, Alzheimer's disease, and basically a terrible life. I'm sure these scientists meant to raise awareness for the importance of sleep, but the results for me, and many others, were far from positive. I totally bought into the fact that sleep was the single biggest factor getting in the way of my health, and that I could not get even one bad night of sleep or else my life would be in shambles. Thus, after a couple months of getting the best sleep of my life, my sleep proceeded to suck for about two months. Every night I would get in bed, dread a poor night of sleep, and toss and turn for hours, some nights not getting more than 2 hours of sleep despite lying down for 8.

Since their rise to stardom, these scientists have been deeply scrutinized for their claims. Thankfully, I became aware of these criticisms and learned that sleep anxiety was indeed a real problem. I learned that the doomsday-like claims made by some of these well-meaning scientists were a stretch, at best. If you struggle with sleep anxiety, I urge you to focus on how incredibly resilient the body is. Approach sleep with humility—even the most prestigious scientists do not fully know how the body makes such remarkable repairs to our body during sleep. What do I mean by that? *Let go* of trying to force a good night of sleep and let your body take control—it knows best. And remember: one night of poor sleep will not make or break your life.

CHAPTER 6: NUTRITION, METABOLISM, AND MICROBES—THE CONTROL CENTERS FOR IMMUNITY

"All disease begins in the gut" - Hippocrates

It's no secret that nutrition is at the core of our health. What we eat is broken down into the building blocks which make up our cell membranes, proteins, and molecular machinery. Food fuels every chemical reaction which sustains us.

As I came to learn more about the inner workings of modern medicine, I came to realize that it's normal to think of the human body like the interior of a car. The windshield doesn't affect the steering wheel. But for the body, that's often not the case. The body seems to be an interconnected system—disease in one area of the body probably means disease/dysfunction in at least one other part of the body. This is exactly the case with metabolic dysfunction. In fact, as the data have rolled in, scientists can now comfortably make a shocking claim: *"The major risk factor for severe COVID-19 is poor metabolic health,*" [174].

What the heck is metabolic health? A recent study titled "Prevalence of Optimal Metabolic Health in American Adults: National Health and Nutrition Examination Survey 2009-2016", researchers found that among the general population, only about 12% of Americans are *metabolically healthy*. Metabolism refers to the way the body uses and stores energy. Considering fasting blood glucose, HbA1c, insulin, cholesterol, and waist circumference, only a tiny fraction of Americans are deemed to be metabolically healthy[175]. The shocking part is, *even healthy-looking people* may not fall into the category of metabolically healthy. In fact, in the study, more than two-thirds of *normal weight adults* were metabolically unhealthy.

How is that specifically relevant to COVID-19? Due to chronic inflammation, which is a hallmark of obesity, the risk of *many* diseases increases[176]:

- High blood pressure, type 2 diabetes, cardiovascular disease, and stroke[177]
- Several cancers[178]
- Mental illness[179]
- All-cause mortality (basically, increased risk of death from all causes)[180]
- Severe COVID-19

It's important to realize that almost all of these conditions *independently* lead to worse COVID-19 outcomes regardless of weight status[181]. Now remember that the U.S. adult obesity rate is *just shy* of 50%[182]. Not only are obese individuals more likely to have a severe case of COVID-19, but they also tend to shed the virus significantly more, making them very good at spreading it. Researchers note: "...*all volunteers of <26 y of age and all subjects under 22 BMI were low* *spreaders of exhaled bioaerosol… 18% of human subjects (35) accounted for 80% of the exhaled bioaerosol of the group (194),"* [183]. What does that mean? Obese and metabolically unhealthy people seem to be the "superspreaders", responsible for most (80%) of the spread of COVID-19. On the other hand, young and healthy people are responsible for significantly less transmission. Unfortunately, there was little mention of this issue in the media. If it would have been mentioned, maybe this would have given people the motivation to seek out help, change their habits, and transform their lives. Obviously, obesity is a complex, multifactorial issue, but with proper education, guidance, simple lifestyle modifications, and a strong *why*, this condition is, by no means, permanent.

Now, let's talk about the gut. Your gut does *much* more than simply break down food. Often referred to as the second brain for its connections to the brain, the gut is also responsible for regulating our mood, metabolism, and is *critical for our immune health.* The signals between the immune system and gut are collectively known as *Immune-microbe crosstalk.* Immune-microbe crosstalk is simply a fancy term for the way the microbes in our gut talk to the immune system. Just how important is this crosstalk? About 80% of your immune system is found in the gut. But it doesn't end there. The composition of your gut microbiome—the collection of trillions of bacteria, fungi, and archaea—affects our risk of developing autoimmune diseases, obesity, type 2 diabetes, cancer, Crohn's disease, and several other diseases[184]. Our gut microbes can also defend against bacterial infections by "crowding out," or directly inhibiting the growth of, harmful, pathogenic bacteria. They do this by secreting antimicrobial substances and competing for resources[185]. More recently, the gut microbiota has also been shown to affect our susceptibility to *viral infections*. A review paper published in the journal *Immunological Reviews,* gave three possible situations: "*The host's microbiota can potentially influence viral infections in three ways: their presence could be neutral, their presence could hinder viral infection, or their presence could promote viral infection,*" [186]. The gut microbiome has been shown to influence how well our immune system can defend against influenza infections[187]. It can also influence the rate at which viruses replicate[188]! Uncontrolled viral replication may be one of the reasons for severe infections[189].

By now, a common theme throughout this book should be that virtually every part of the body affects every other part of the body. Recently, the discovery of the "gut-lung axis" has confirmed this idea. How does the gut "talk" to the lungs? *Endotoxins* (which are pro-inflammatory), cytokines, and other gut microbiome-derived substances can influence the function of the lungs[190]. Indeed, gut microbes have been found to influence the *lung's susceptibility to viral infections[191]*. More research has shown that dysbiosis— imbalance of "good" and "bad" bacteria in the gut— leads to more severe asthma in animals[192]. Some studies have shown similar results in humans. Reduced abundance of the species *Akkermansia muciniphila* and *Faecalibacterium prausnitzii* have been found in children with asthma compared to those without asthma[193].

So, it's pretty clear by now that the gut microbiome is involved in lung function as well as immune response to the flu. But how does it relate to COVID-19 specifically? Research now suggests that the composition of the gut microbiome predicts

COVID-19 severity. By now, it is well known that an overactive, hyper-inflammatory immune response to the virus is largely what determines severity[194]. A study published in the journal *Gut* by the *British Medical Journal* studied the stool and blood of 100 COVID-19-positive patients and found exactly that. In addition to heightened inflammatory markers (IL-6, CRP, etc.), patients with severe COVID-19 also demonstrated higher levels of *Bacteroidetes,* lower levels of *Actinobacteria,* and lower levels of the generally anti-inflammatory *Faecalibacterium prausnitzii* and *Bifidobacterium bifidum*[195]. In plain English, the makeup of the gut bacteria predicted the degree of inflammatory immune response to SARS-CoV-2! This does not necessarily mean you should go out and try to stock up on probiotics with these species. The world of probiotic supplements is very complex and often disappointing. Despite what many gut health gurus claim, scientists still debate the idea that there is *one* specific "healthy" microbiome or microbe *everyone* should aim to have. As some scientists put it, *"Health effects of specific microbiome features might well be* **context dependent, and bacterial taxa being associated with health in one disease setting and disease in another have already been reported"** [196]. In other words, myopically searching for and targeting that *one* perfect gut microbe species might be narrow-minded and does not yet have sufficient evidence to support it.

So, how can you keep your gut healthy to support immune health and reduce your risk of developing disease? And how can you support your metabolic health to do the same?

Eat Whole Foods—with an Emphasis on Protein

Eating a wide range of whole foods (basically, limiting anything processed or in a box) is the simplest way to increase your intake of crucial vitamins and minerals (micronutrients) without having to dish out hundreds of dollars for expensive supplements. The expensive supplements to consider are icing on the cake once the foundation (eating real food) is implemented. But eating whole foods aren't just a way to increase micronutrient status. Whole foods—plant and animal foods—tend to be more fibrous, have more water content, and are more *satiating*. This inevitably leads one to eat less food, improve metabolic health, and maintain a healthy weight more effortlessly. On the other hand, following the Standard American Diet (SAD)—high in low-quality fats and refined carbohydrates at the expense of protein—leads to overconsumption of calories, and therefore, weight gain[197]. This is known as the protein leverage hypothesis, where, due to protein's high satiety (it makes you feel full), you tend to eat less food more effortlessly, without relying solely on willpower.

While going from eating processed foods to eating a wide variety of whole foods (plants or animals) will be beneficial for virtually everyone, let's talk about what's optimal in terms of nutrient density and bioavailability. While I know this may anger some vegan and plant-based zealots, animal products generally have the highest nutrient density and *bioavailability*—the nutrients are absorbed and used more easily by our bodies[198]. Contrary to popular belief, animal foods aren't just fat and protein. Not only are these foods a better source of the *active* forms of vitamins (preformed vitamin A, D3, and K2), creatine, carnitine, zinc, DHA, and choline, but they're also more *bioavailable* when compared to plant foods[199]. In other words, if you pit a plant food versus an animal food with the same amount of calcium, for example, you will tend to absorb more calcium from the meat than the plant. From my understanding it seems that humans evolved eating a large amount of meat and this is partially what led to the evolution of our giant brains, acidic stomachs, and small guts[200]. I promise I'm not paid by the meat and dairy industry—trust me, as a college student, I kind of wish I was. Anyway, much to the dismay of vegan Karens, animal products simply seem to be superior in terms of nutrient density and bioavailability. If you really want optimal nutrient density, reach for organ meats—liver, kidney, heart, etc. These foods have been prized since early humans began scavenging and hunting animals. Add some seasonal fruits and vegetables to it and that's really as simple as a diet needs to be.

That's not to say you can't do well on a plant-based diet if you really want to do so. Let me explain. For most of human history, humans have used technology to enhance nutrient availability, neutralize plant defenses, and make food more easily digestible. In the past few centuries, however, humans have used technology to make food hyper-palatable, increase profit margins, and give processed food a near-unlimited shelf life. What's the problem? If you choose to eat a plant-based diet, at least take some wisdom from our ancestors, and make these foods more nutritious and bioavailable by sprouting, soaking, and fermenting foods. If you want more information on ancestral food preparation, Dr. Bill Schindler, one of my previous podcast guests, is the man. You can check out the episode I did with him, as well as his book "Eat Like a Human" to learn more.

Natural Birth Beats C-section

This section probably feels a bit out of place in a chapter mostly focused on nutrition. But since we're talking about microbes, and I mentioned that Mr. Average Joe was born via c-section, I thought I'd explain why that's important. Concurrent with the epidemics of autoimmune diseases, there has been a huge surge in the rate of cesarean section surgeries. According to the United States Department of Health and Human Services (HHS), ~32% of deliveries are c-section[201]. How exactly does the mode of delivery affect long-term health outcomes? It is theorized that the gut microbiome is "seeded" during a critical period after birth. In other words, you are not born with the microbiome you have now. Therefore, the first microbes to which babies are exposed, *take over*, or colonize, their guts. Naturally, the vaginal microbiome should provide these fundamental microbes for the baby. Bypassing this process, however, does not allow the baby's microbiome to be properly "seeded," and subsequently can lead to abnormal development of the immune system. In fact, several studies have shown that babies delivered by c-section are more likely to develop autoimmune conditions, food allergies[202] and are at an increased risk of gastrointestinal conditions[203].

Trust me I wish it weren't true. As a c-section baby myself, I now know I probably missed out on a peak gut microbiome from not being born naturally. Obviously, in many cases, c-section is the only way to go if the baby's or the mother's life is on the line. However, that doesn't negate the potential negative effects of bypassing the vaginal microbiome. I want to be clear that I'm not telling you this to further worry you and create a nocebo effect, where thinking about the fact that you didn't come out of your mother's vagina means that you will lead a terrible life. No. As someone who can be quite obsessive about health, I know how much it sucks to think yourself into worse health because *someone* said *something* is bad for you and you believed them. Instead, I tell you this because knowledge is power—the hard part is learning how to wield it. Otherwise stated, this section should hopefully bring your awareness to the fact that, perhaps a disturbed microbiome *could be a place to further explore* if you were born via c-section and are suffering with an autoimmune disease, depression, anxiety, or another condition affected by the gut microbiome[204].

Skip the Drink

Yes, probably even the organic, biodynamic, fair trade, dry wine. Sorry. A paper published in *The Lancet* titled "No level of alcohol consumption improves health" requires no further explanation on my part[205]. Alcohol has been shown to significantly increase the risk of acute respiratory distress syndrome—a major severe complication from COVID-19[206]. If you read no other part of this book, alcohol alone makes it quite clear that the risk of severe COVID-19 is not just "Russian Roulette". Alcohol consumption also increases the risk of almost every major chronic disease which plagues mankind today, including heart disease, cancer, depression, epilepsy, stroke, liver damage, and the list goes on and on[207]. It's important to note that virtually all of these diseases *independently* increase the risk of severe COVID-19. It's amazing that the stuff is legal, but not psilocybin mushrooms or marijuana. Makes sense.

Anyways, before you hurl your empty wine bottle at me, just know that I get it—the pandemic led to a worldwide depression. We didn't have our friends, our family, our jobs, and our normal way of life. For many of those who do not have the resources to get a therapist or take the time to take care of your health, the most easily available sources of pleasure were undoubtedly drugs, food, and alcohol. In fact, it was *not food,* but rather alcohol consumption which was the major downfall amongst my health coaching clients which led to dramatic weight gain (20+ pounds) during the pandemic. Over a year of social isolation was either an opportunity to change your life radically or a time when health got dramatically worse… For many people, the latter was true—and alcohol absolutely played a major role.

Of course, quality of life matters too, right? I'm a college student—I *know* how much people like their alcohol. Therefore, it's unrealistic to ask people to permanently give up a drink every now and then—in that case a reasonable serving of the aforementioned wine would probably be your best choice. But the way I see it, a *foundation* of good health should be built before indulging every once in a while—at least, if you care about your health.

Magnesium

As I've already explained, magnesium is an essential mineral which many Americans do not get enough of. Magnesium supplementation has been shown to help moderately improve scores of insulin resistance (the hallmark of type 2 diabetes), improve insulin sensitivity[208], and reduce fasting blood sugar in people with high blood sugar[209]. Magnesium also seems to play a role in inflammation, with deficiencies increasing oxidative stress, Interleukin-6 (IL-6), and C-reactive protein[210]. As I explained earlier, IL-6 is a cytokine associated with inflammation and a "cytokine storm", which is theorized to be responsible for severe COVID-19. Highly sensitive C-reactive protein (hsCRP) is another common measure of inflammation elevated in people with obesity, Alzheimer's disease[211], heart disease, and—you guessed it—severe COVID-19[212]. Therefore, adequate magnesium intake may indirectly lower the risk of severe COVID-19 by improving metabolic health and decreasing inflammation in those who do not get enough magnesium.

In addition, magnesium has been found to be important in directly modulating the immune system. It seems to play an important role in regulating natural killer cells as well as T cells, both of which are important in fighting an infection and forming a lasting immune response. It should come as no surprise that a magnesium deficiency has been found to lead to immunosuppression[213].

Cut Out Sugar

Cutting out refined carbohydrates and added sugar may be one of the simplest steps to improve health mainly because it's easy to overconsume sugar. Doing so chronically leads to high blood sugar, triglycerides, and insulin. Although chronically high blood sugar has very clearly been shown to be deleterious to health, even short bouts of sky-high blood sugar have been shown to worsen immune health[214].

Replace refined carbohydrate sources with *whole foods* instead. Instead of a piece of white bread, eat some unsweetened yogurt with berries. Rather than munching on pretzels, have a piece of 80% dark chocolate sweetened with stevia. There are endless alternatives to these refined products—you just have to be willing to look and experiment.

The Importance of Insulin

Let's begin with insulin. Insulin is a crucial hormone which allows glucose into cells. Every time you eat a meal, blood sugar rises, leading to a rise in insulin to store as fat or burn it. This is great when it comes to returning our blood sugar to normal after a meal. However, when this mechanism is overused and abused, it becomes a problem.

Following a long-term pattern of overeating can lead to hyperinsulinemia (chronically high insulin). This condition is associated with numerous health conditions, including Alzheimer's disease, magnesium deficiency, obesity, type 2 diabetes, lower vitamin D status, cancer, and heart disease[215,216]. Hyperinsulinemia also increases oxidative stress, abnormal blood clotting, and pulmonary embolism (a blood clot which gets lodged in a lung artery)[217].

So, if you're someone who tends to overeat on a regular basis, try the following: make unsweetened tea; have a glass of water; ask yourself why you want to snack. Is it hunger driven or emotionally driven? Is it a distraction? Empty stimulation? Switch out mindless snacking for another feel-good task. Try reading, working out, listening to music, going for a walk, exercising, spending time with family, or calling a friend.

Feeding the Gut

Most people have heard of the foods which contain "good bacteria": Kimchi, kefir, sauerkraut, and yogurt (just watch out for added sugars). These foods are rich in *probiotics*—actual living microbes which can replenish the gut microbiome. As with everything in this book, there are few blanket statements about nutrition because health really is an individual matter. Fermented foods could be a double-edged sword. They contain a high amount of *histamine,* which is not well tolerated by those with histamine intolerance (discussed in depth soon). I'd recommend keeping a food journal to see how you feel after each meal to see if you might be sensitive to specific foods. I digress.

The previous foods are sources of bacteria, but what about the microbes? What do they eat? *Prebiotics.* Soluble fibers, such as ß-glucans, pectin, and resistant starch, are actually broken down by our gut bacteria, since we can't digest it ourselves[218]. These fuels allow bacteria to create a fuel known as Short Chain Fatty Acids (SCFAs). Why are SCFAs important? They seem to be important in reducing inflammation. How? Stay with me. There are two main categories of macrophages (a type of white blood cell): M1 (inflammatory) and M2 (anti-inflammatory). A SCFA called *butyrate* seems to be able to shift macrophages to the anti-inflammatory version, M2[219]. Let's put it all together: eating prebiotic fibers from vegetables and seasonal fruits feeds the gut bacteria, allowing them to produce SCFAs and shift macrophages towards the *anti-inflammatory* version. In some animal models, it has already been shown that consumption of prebiotic fibers are able to protect against influenza infection[220]. Theoretically, targeting butyrate production could be an important preventative strategy against the cytokine storm.

In addition, a recent paper done by Stanford University showed that a diet rich in fermented foods (probiotic-rich foods) increased microbial diversity in the gut, as well as *decreased* levels of interleukin 6 (IL-6)[221]. The link between IL-6 and severe COVID-19 is so strong, that the World Health Organization is now recommending the use of interleukin-6 receptor *blockers* to lessen severity of COVID-19[222]! Therefore, slowly introducing fermented foods and fiber-rich foods into your diet seems to be a good strategy to improve gut health and decrease inflammation.

Histamine

If you're a diet fanatic, hopping around from one hot trend to the next, you've likely heard of the low histamine diet. If you have an allergy, you've probably taken an *antihistamine* to clear up the congestion, itchiness, skin sensitivity, headache, and inflammation. But what is histamine and why would you want less of it? Histamine is a substance found in high amounts in the gut, lungs, and skin—specifically in the mast cells (a type of white blood cell). We make histamine ourselves, but we can also find it in foods. Histamine has been found to regulate inflammation, *cytokines*, and the immune response[223]. Histamine is theorized to initiate, "...*abnormal immune response leading to cytokine storm and multi-organs failure,*" [224]. Specifically, a disorder known as Mast Cell Activation Syndrome (MCAS) involves overactive mast cells which produce excess histamine and promote too much inflammation[225].

MCAS has been estimated to affect almost 20% of people living in first-world nations. In fact, one compelling theory which explains why some may experience a cytokine storm, and therefore, a severe reaction to COVID-19, is the presence of dysfunctional mast cells. Remember back to my earlier rant about how not being overtly sick doesn't mean you are actually healthy? Turns out, this is extremely relevant to patients with MCAS: "*...most MCAS patients remain undiagnosed and untreated, and therefore their dysfunctional MCs, whether causing mild or severe illness, are uncontrolled and may react inappropriately to SARS-CoV-2...* **many MCAS patients who have been undiagnosed for decades tend to minimise their problems, sometimes deceivingly declaring themselves as 'healthy',**" [226].

To be clear, this does not mean "histamine bad". What it seems to imply is that an *imbalance* of histamine, *at the wrong times,* and *for an abnormal duration* is problematic. But how is it relevant to COVID-19? One review article discussed the efficacy of histamine blocker famotidine in reducing risk of death from COVID-19 by 32.5%; combining aspirin and famotidine had a synergistic effect[227].

What affects histamine levels in the body? For starters, your genetics can play a role in abnormally high histamine levels. Enzymes necessary for breaking down histamine may be "slow", leading to a buildup of histamine[228]. In addition, certain foods can be problematic. The most straightforward way of reducing the amount of histamine in your body is by reducing dietary intake of histamine-rich foods, such as pineapple, bananas, citrus fruits, fermented foods, alcohol, and tomatoes. Other factors such as mold[229] and excess endurance exercise[230] can increase histamine in the body. Remember, health and nutrition are usually not one-size-fits-all recommendations. What is a health food for one person could be an inflammatory food for another person.

What can be done? Natural antihistamines, such as quercetin or vitamin C[231] can be found in foods such as onions, fresh vegetables, and fruits. Several opinion pieces and review articles hypothesize that they would be helpful in COVID-19 treatment due to quercetin's antihistamine and anti-inflammatory effects[232]. In addition, quercetin is a zinc ionophore, meaning that it helps your body absorb zinc into your cells more readily, which could theoretically help zinc do its job better. Zinc, is important in reducing viral replication, improving natural killer cell activity, and being anti-inflammatory[233]. I took quercetin and zinc as supplements when I had COVID-19 and found it very helpful for congestion. However, to my knowledge, no studies have been done with COVID-19 and quercetin alone.

Finally, it's also important to note that just because a news article says "Supplement X does/does not work for COVID-19" you *really* have to look beyond the headline. The timing, dosage, and interactions with other compounds greatly impact the efficacy of a supplement. Always, always, *always* seek context when black or white statements are hurled at you. If you choose to start supplementing, it is always wise to speak with your doctor to see if certain compounds could interact with medications.

I recommend checking out my episode with Dr. Tina Peers on this topic to learn more.

Yet Another Controversy in Nutrition: What are Good Fats?

When I first began writing this section, I have to admit that I blindly believed the health gurus who claimed that vegetable and seed oils—such as canola, grapeseed, corn, safflower, and soybean oils—were to blame for virtually every chronic disease known to man. What I found as I dug into the scientific literature, however, revealed a different, more nuanced, story.

The health effects of vegetable oils are controversial partially because they are high in omega-6, polyunsaturated fats (PUFAs). The anti-omega-6 crowd claims that high consumption of PUFAs and omega 6 fats have been shown to be highly inflammatory. Consumption of vegetable oils, and specifically linoleic acid, are hypothesized to increase risk of cardiovascular disease[234]. Other research suggests that *repeatedly heating* these unstable vegetable oils can lead to unwanted chemical byproducts, since the oil becomes oxidized and, therefore, dangerous[235]. In addition, the ratio of omega 6 to omega 3 fat intake seems to be important for health. Several studies have suggested that when fats rich in omega 3 were substituted for omega 6-rich oils, lower levels of inflammation were found[236]. What seems to be most true in this argument is the fact that the ratio of dietary omega 6 to omega 3 fats is, at least somewhat, important[237]. Unsurprisingly, the Standard American Diet ensures a ridiculously high intake of omega 6 compared to omega 3. The ratio our ancestors ate, according to anthropological research, is estimated to be around 1:1, whereas the standard American diet is now estimated to be at least 15:1[238].

Now, for the other side of the story. There are

some *major* studies which show no effect[239] or a positive health effect[240] on heart disease or mortality from consuming omega 6 fats—specifically linoleic acid which often tends to be vilified. As always, the truth is probably somewhere in the middle… *But*, I'll explain later on why I still stay far away from omega 6-rich oils.

Before I do that, let's talk about saturated fats. As I explained in the beginning of this book, evidence has been steadily mounting which states that not only is there little correlation between saturated fat intake[241] and coronary artery disease or mortality[242], but some research even suggests a lower risk of stroke[243, 244] with higher consumption of saturated fat instead of vegetable oils[245]. Needless to say, many researchers are beginning to question the long-held belief that unsaturated fats and/or vegetable oils are *always* better than saturated fat[246].

As with virtually *everything,* the research is not totally clear and also depends on your genetics. Out of precaution, I mostly cook with avocado and olive oil, *rarely* with grass fed butter, Ghee, coconut oil, grass-fed tallow, and lard from pastured pork, and *never* with vegetable oils. Why?

Although the literature does not fully support the idea that seed oils are to blame for all of mankind's problems, that does not mean seed oils are innocent. We must remember that time and time again "*the science*" has been wrong—it just takes *years* for new evidence to usurp an old dogma. So, despite the murky research, I still stay *far* away from these oils (well, as much as I can in a college dining hall). Why? Think of a soybean—not much fat on there, huh? How do you suppose someone could mass produce tons of oil from a lean soybean? Just squeeze it with your fingers until oil comes oozing out of its pores? Wishful thinking. In order to get any usable oil from a soybean, you must put a *huge* quantity of them under high pressure and heat. It doesn't end there, however. The byproduct of this first step is a foggy-looking, putrid-smelling substance which must be treated with a chemical solvent (often petroleum-based) to get rid of the foul smell and appearance. Heart healthy? I don't buy it, but again this is just my opinion using the precautionary principle and common sense.

Leaky Gut

Considered pseudoscience by conventional medicine until recently, intestinal permeability (leaky gut) seems to be a detriment to immune health. So, what is leaky gut?

Think of your intestinal lining as a zipper. When the epithelial cells of the gut (the teeth of the zipper) are working properly, they are *tightly held together* by tight junctions, only allowing certain substances through. Why does it work this way? The proximal answer is: eating food means taking a foreign substance into the body and trying to assimilate it. So, there may be *bacteria, toxins, or other potentially harmful substances* within the food we consume. These tight junctions serve to protect you from having those dangerous substances enter the bloodstream.

In the case of leaky gut, however, this system is broken. The gut lining is torn or swollen, leaving the zipper wide open to foreign substances. Why is this an issue for immune health? Gut dysbiosis is likely to occur when leaky gut is present. Dysbiosis basically means an imbalance of gut microbes, which interferes with: production of neurotransmitters, regulation of antioxidant defenses, metabolism regulation, and cognitive health—all of which are crucial for proper immunity. Leaky gut usually comes hand in hand with bloating, digestive issues, brain fog, autoimmune conditions, and more[247].

There are many different ways to combat this issue. Here are some of them:

- *Fasting.* Fasting can be thought of as a break for the digestive system. This allows the body to use energy for other bodily processes, upregulated *autophagy* being the most well-known benefit—although calorie restriction (eating less throughout the day) can accomplish the same. "Auto-phagy", or self-eating, allows the body to clear out and recycle damaged proteins and cellular debris. Fasting has been shown to specifically improve gut barrier function[248]. When fasting is combined with other protocols, it can be very helpful for improving gut health and digestion.

- *Bone broth... again.* The high amount of collagen and glycine in bone broth make it great for gut health. In fact, research has demonstrated a protective effect of collagen intake on gut integrity. You do not necessarily need to consume bone broth, however. You can take a supplement, such as a grass-fed collagen peptides powder[249].

- *Limiting wheat consumption.* Today's wheat is a totally different animal than the wheat our ancestors ate. Basically, the modern wheat crop has been ridiculously modified over the past few years. It has mainly been modified and selected to be resistant to pesticides and produce massive crop yields. In doing so, it has also given us much less time to adapt to this new form of wheat—known as *dwarf wheat*. In addition, the presence of gluten, gliadin, agglutinin, and other plant defenses have been shown to be deleterious to the integrity of the gut lining[250, 251]. As with everything, *you* may not have a problem with wheat, while your brother, sister, or mom might—pay attention to how you react to foods. If you're a bread lover like I am, one way to neutralize some of the plant defenses and make wheat more digestible is to make slow-fermented sourdough bread.

- *Soaking and sprouting raw nuts, legumes, and seeds.* Since plants cannot run from us, they've developed their own chemical defense systems[252]. These are called antinutrients, such as phytates, lectins, and oxalates which could wreak havoc on the gut, depending on your individual sensitivities and gut health[253]. Soaking and sprouting foods reduces the content of these potentially harmful plant defenses, increasing digestibility and the availability of nutrients.

Eating Local

We've often heard that eating local is good for the environment, for supporting local farms, and for getting your hands on fresh food. While those are all true, there's something much more fascinating about eating food which grows in your immediate environment.

If you've gotten this far, you likely already know this, but it is worth reiterating: our world is a microbe-driven world. In fact, there are more microbes living within us than cells in our bodies. No "germs" means no life. How does this relate to local eating?

Let's say you live in the northern hemisphere––cold winters and hot summers. Now, think about what kinds of foods would be available if grocery stores were nonexistent. In the summer, you'd find a small variety of fruits—likely some berries, cherries, and peaches. In the winter, you'd find much less variety—some lettuce, carrots, and root vegetables. What you will not find in northern Canada, for example, is a mango tree growing in the backyard. This may not be a trivial occurrence. Let me explain. Local eating *equals* seasonal eating. Food type and availability vary with the seasons. How does that affect the microbiome? Since certain foods feed certain microbes in your body, the *types* (diversity) and *amounts* (richness) of microbes *also change* from season to season. In fact, stool samples from the Hadza showed changes to microbial diversity and richness depending on whether it was dry season (animal-based diet) or wet season (plant-based diet). This change is an adaptation which promote certain gut bacteria, allowing them to digest season-specific foods better, and enter a sort of homeostasis with the environment[254]. Although there are no studies to my knowledge which show *exactly* what this means in terms of health, I think it's worth thinking about. It seems that most of the things we have considered trivial (pesticides, artificial light, hyper-sterile homes, c-section, etc.) come to bite us in the butt years later. It's possible that seasonal eating, along with a seasonal change in the gut microbiome, may have some effect on our health.

Algae

Yup, you read that right. Algae, as I learned just last year, is not just for whales. Specifically, I'm going to be discussing *spirulina*, a blue-green algae which has been of great interest to NASA and the United Nations alike. While, at first, I believed spirulina to be just another fringe vegan supplement, I now recognize its profound nutritional, and even medicinal, value. Spirulina has thousands of studies which discuss its antimicrobial, antioxidant, anti-inflammatory[255], weight loss[256] and immunomodulating[257] effects.

In fact, spirulina and spirulina-derived compounds are being studied as therapies for COVID-19. Phycocyanobilins, sulphate polysaccharides, and other compounds all found in spirulina, could be potent antivirals against SARS-CoV2[258]. Additionally, SARS-CoV2 gets into cells via the ACE2 receptor. Spirulina has been found to work as an ACE-inhibitor which could theoretically lead to less severity, although this is not yet clinically proven. Regardless of the interaction between spirulina and ACE receptors, *"Spirulina nutraceuticals and derived ACE inhibitory peptides have been well demonstrated to **boost immune response, reduction in cytokine-related inflammation, and enhancing ACE2 activity** in in vitro, in vivo, and in silico studies on model animal organisms and humans in different diseases"* [259].

Finally, spirulina is nutrient-dense. Loaded with B-vitamins, chlorophyll, vitamin A, vitamin K and beyond, algae seems to be one of the few foods that actually deserve the title of a superfood. I basically use it as a natural multivitamin when I'm traveling, and I recommend it to anyone looking to upgrade their nutrition in a convenient way.

Organic

Earlier, I shared the fact that glyphosate led to gut microbiome dysbiosis—essentially killing some of the beneficial bacteria, allowing the harmful bacteria to proliferate[260, 261]. Why does this matter? In a healthy gut microbiome, microbes produce powerful *antiviral* compounds[262]. Since gut microbiome health *directly* controls immune health, dysbiosis is a *clear detriment* to the body's ability to handle viruses properly. In addition, non-Hodgkin's lymphoma (NHL), a white blood cell cancer, is strongly linked to glyphosate[263]. In fact, scientists estimate that a previously reported 41% increase in NHL—in people chronically exposed to glyphosate—is likely an *underestimate[264]*.

One of the common arguments for glyphosate being safe is the idea that "The dose makes the poison". While true, what this argument often misses is the fact that we are not just exposed to glyphosate in our food, but also in the water we drink and the air we breathe, which means that we're getting a much larger dose of herbicides than we think. Regardless, some scientists are taking the side of the EPA, arguing that Roundup is only toxic at very high doses[265].

Unlike other natural health advocates, I don't think non-organic food is the root of all disease. Like all subjects discussed in this book, there are always two sides to every story. Obviously, I'm not an expert in this field, but I know enough to say that there *are* experts on both sides of the debate. It would be a disservice to you if I didn't acknowledge that.

As often as possible, I choose organic foods. Fortunately, my family is in a situation where we can afford them. **I want to be very clear that if you are** not in a financial situation to buy wildly expensive organic food, eating unprocessed conventional food is still better than processed food! This all-or-nothing, hyper-perfectionistic mindset perpetuated by many health gurus is not helpful in the real world.

Start a Garden
Starting your own garden is a simple way to get around the expense or availability of organic foods. I recommend you check out Farmer's Footprint, an amazing organization dedicated to converting farms from commercial farming to regenerative agriculture. Learn how to grow your own garden—even if you live in a small apartment or in a city—at https://farmersfootprint.us/resources/.

The Simple Things No One Wants to Hear
Exercise, get good sleep, manage stress, and eat whole foods. Again, rather than trying to focus on targeting a specific microbe, turn your attention to the things which will give you the biggest bang for your buck. For example, exercise has been shown to positively impact the composition of the gut microbiome[266]. Same idea with stress—having overwhelming psychological stress can influence your gut microbiota via inflammatory signaling molecules and hormones[267]. Therefore, getting the big stuff right will have the greatest impact on health—everything past that is icing on the cake.

RESOURCES AND FURTHER READING

1. Dr. Marvin Singh

2. Dr. Tom Bayne
3. Dr. Ben Bikman
4. Dr. James Dinicolantonio
5. Dr. Layne Norton
6. Dr. Chris Masterjohn
7. Dr. Peter Attia
8. Dr. Chris Kresser
9. Dr. Aseem Malhotra
10. Dr. Pran Yoganathan
11. *The Yoga of Eating* by Charles Eisenstein
12. Dr. Zach Bush
13. Dr. William Davis
14. Catharine Arnston

CHAPTER 7: LIGHT SHAPES LIFE

15 minutes. That's how long it used to take for me to get a sunburn. I know—pretty pathetic. My fate was clear: I would forever be stuck with pasty white skin and I needed to continuously cower from the sun. Or so I thought. Growing up, I had measly vitamin D levels, which reflected the fact that I couldn't be outside for longer than 15 minutes without turning into a lobster. If you're unfamiliar with vitamin D levels, below 30 ng/ml is considered by many to be a deficiency. Since I was 3 points higher than a deficiency, it was never an issue for my doctor. So, I went about most of my childhood and adolescence unaware that I was missing this powerful compound for hormonal health, sleep, and *immune health*.

About a year ago, I learned a lesson from several of my podcast guests: not deficient doesn't mean optimal. In other words, there's a spectrum of vitamin D levels, conferring different health benefits for different diseases. Take breast cancer for example. The lowest risk of developing breast cancer is seen at vitamin D levels greater than or equal to 60ng/ml—far above the threshold for a deficiency. As your levels go up from a deficiency, certain health markers of health improve (up until a certain point). Empowered by this new knowledge, I made it a point to go outside as often as possible. What many dermatologists and doctors did not tell me was that there was emerging evidence of vitamin D's role as anti-cancer[268, 269]. While *consistently* getting a *sunburn* increases the risk of developing melanoma (skin cancer), long term occupational sun exposure was not related to the development of melanoma[270]. Why? Well, it could be due to the natural rise in vitamin D levels as you *gradually* spend more time in the sun.

In addition, melanin, which is produced in response to sun exposure and makes your skin darker, protects against sun exposure. Melanin has been shown to decrease the spread of melanoma[271] and is now widely known to decrease the risk of developing melanoma in the first place[272]. Of course, based on our individual ancestry and genetics, we have a different capacity for producing melanin (I'll explain how I navigate sun exposure with limited melanin production). But I think it's still pretty amazing. Mother nature had mechanisms to protect us from the harsh rays of the sun—yet another example of the fact that our body isn't stupid. Before the advent of modern sunscreen and chemotherapy, I sincerely doubt that all hunter-gatherers were walking tumors.

Nitric Oxide

Nitric Oxide (N.O.) is a compound released as UV rays strike the skin[273]. As a powerful vasodilator (dilates blood vessels), it increases blood flow and reduces blood pressure. However, that's not all N.O. does. N.O. also acts to stop viruses from replicating! Here is some of what is known about nitric oxide's role in immunity:

"N.O. is important as a toxic defense molecule against infectious organisms. It also regulates the functional activity, growth and death of many immune and inflammatory cell types including macrophages, T lymphocytes, antigen-presenting cells, mast cells, neutrophils and natural killer cells," [274]. N.O. seems to directly be antimicrobial and is involved in regulating cells critical to our immune response.

"Viral replication is inhibited by the induction of iNOS and the subsequent production of NO," [275].

"Nitric oxide (NO) produced by the airway epithelium is vital to antiviral inflammatory and immune defense in the lung," [276]. With so much talk of ventilators early in the pandemic, it became increasingly clear that lung failure played a role in severe COVID-19 cases. In this regard, proper nitric oxide levels seem to be important.

Sunlight Exposure and Our Circadian Rhythms

Recently, the study of circadian rhythms, the 24-hour cycle of sleep/wake in humans, has grown exponentially. It is now well known that the type and intensity of light we are exposed to throughout the day is an important signal to the body. This is known as a *zeitgeber*, or time giver. Basically, light tells our body, via our eyes and skin, what time of day it is. In response to this information, our body releases certain hormones and neurotransmitters at the right times of day: cortisol and testosterone peaks in the morning; melatonin peaks at night. However, if you are exposed to bright light at night, it sends the wrong signals to the body, disrupting the normal circadian rhythm. Like I discussed in the chapter on sleep, disrupting sleep consistently is detrimental to immune health.

Slow and Steady

Although the benefits of sunlight are undeniable, ultraviolet radiation (UVR) can do some damage. The real damage comes from deciding to spend hours in the sun all at once after years of living an indoor lifestyle. Here's where some common sense is necessary. Exposing yourself to the sun *before* you get a sunburn is typically a good way to build up solar resilience. Start slow and allow your skin to adapt to increased sunlight exposure. You'll probably notice that you'll burn less, tan more, and be able to stay out for longer.

To Vitamin D and Beyond

The conversation surrounding vitamin D has been somewhat controversial this year. To be fair, COVID-19 made virtually everything controversial. I'd argue, however, that there is now enough evidence to show that vitamin D can reduce severity *and* death from COVID-19.

Let me begin with a shocking statistic. A landmark study published in the *British Medical Journal* estimated that, "*9.4% of **all deaths** in Europe and 12.8% of those in the United States could be attributed to vitamin D deficiency,*" [277]. Almost 13% of ALL DEATHS could be traced back to a vitamin D deficiency. Unfortunately, around 40% of U.S. citizens are deficient in vitamin D, with 80% of African Americans and ~70% of Hispanics suffering from a deficiency[278]. However, that 40% is defined as a blood level of 20 ng/ml or lower. Other medical professionals and researchers[279] believe the level should be set significantly higher[280]. Remember, *not deficient* is not the same as *optimal*. In fact, when the threshold of vitamin D is set at 40 ng/ml[281], around 90% of Americans are deficient[282, 283]. But what is it about vitamin D which supports immune health?

Let's begin generally. Before we had direct evidence of vitamin D's effects on COVID-19, what was the evidence for a positive effect of vitamin D on immune function? First, vitamin D has been shown to induce *cathelicidin* (an antibacterial and antiviral polypeptide), reduce autoimmune symptoms, boost mucosal defenses, and reduce excessive inflammation[284]. A deficiency in vitamin D has also been shown to enhance cytokine storms[285], increase risk of Acute Respiratory Distress Syndrome (ARDS)[286], and increase the risk of respiratory infections[287]. Since people mainly die from *complications* from COVID-19 (i.e., pneumonia, respiratory distress, stroke, heart disease, organ failure, etc.), it makes intuitive sense that having adequate vitamin D levels would make the body more resilient, protect against these complications, and thus lead to less hospitalizations and deaths. I would argue that even before we had *direct* evidence—studies specifically looking at vitamin D and COVID-19—we had *sufficient* evidence for the governments and health officials to *at least* mention taking vitamin D preventatively out of pure precaution. But is vitamin D safe enough to recommend without direct evidence for its efficacy in COVID-19? A large review and meta-analysis was published in the *British Medical Journal* in 2017, highlighting the *safety and importance* of vitamin D supplementation in preventing respiratory tract infections[288, 289]. Therefore, due to vitamin D's safety, wide-ranging health benefits, and prevalence of deficiency, I believe it would have been warranted for our health professionals to recommend vitamin D supplementation. Unfortunately, all early public health announcements, at least in the United States, led people to believe they were totally powerless—SARS-CoV-2 was coming for them and all they could do was hide, clean, and stay away from the people they loved. That's not to say that distancing and masks aren't helpful, but claiming that they are the *only* thing people can do is ridiculous and far from "evidence-based".

Now, let's talk about vitamin D and COVID-19 specifically. As the pandemic unfolded, increasing quality and quantity of evidence emerged. Early in the pandemic, several researchers demonstrated correlations between COVID-19 and vitamin D status, with one study finding that 85% of severe COVID-19 patients had a vitamin D deficiency[290]. Unsurprisingly, other research has confirmed that a deficiency in vitamin D significantly increases risk of a severe COVID-19 case[291]. An inverse correlation between C-Reactive Protein and vitamin D levels have also been demonstrated. Why is that important? CRP is considered a proxy for the presence of inflammation––more specifically, a *cytokine* storm. High Vitamin D levels in patients equals lower CRP, lower inflammation, and can lead to a decreased risk of a severe case[292]. Correlations are great, as they oriented scientists towards the possibility that vitamin D would be useful for COVID-19, but they still weren't causal.

As of mid 2021, there is now *causal* evidence for the crucial role vitamin D plays in COVID-19 severity. In early September, the first randomized controlled trial of vitamin D for the treatment of COVID-19 was published[293]. Since then, several others have been published. Researchers in Spain found that treatment with vitamin D virtually extinguishes the risk of requiring intensive care unit (ICU) treatment. In other words, administering vitamin D (in the form of *calcifediol*) meant admission into the ICU was *virtually unnecessary*. Specifically, 50% of *untreated* (no vitamin D) COVID-19 patients were admitted into the ICU, several of whom died. On the other hand, only **2% of patients given vitamin D** required ICU treatment. In those 2%, however, *none died*. Next, vitamin D has not only been shown to reduce mortality and severity (hospitalizations), but it has also been shown to lower your risk of testing positive for COVID-19. While the positivity rate for those with vitamin D levels of under 20 ng/ml was 12.5%, those with levels of 55 ng/ml or higher had a significantly lower rate, at 5.9%[294].

A review on vitamin D and COVID-19 showed that vitamin D's role is still uncertain, partially due to wide variation in methodology—how the patients in each study were treated[295]. Specifically, a trial out of Brazil showed that *one* megadose of vitamin D (200,000 IU!) *10 days after symptom onset* did not decrease hospital stay or severe disease[296]. With all due respect to the researchers, if individuals are checked into the ICU with tanked vitamin D levels, ONE SINGLE dose, no matter how high, is a pathetic approach. Why? A high dose of vitamin D of 100,000 IU (international units), for example, requires ~*7 days* for the vitamin D blood levels to rise and reach their peak. It also only seems to increase on average about 15 ng/ml from baseline[297]. In other words, the Brazil trial caught the patients far too late in their disease to have any meaningful effect. In addition to dosing, *timing* also matters. While supplementing at the point of sickness may not be that helpful according to this trial, the critical missing piece is to supplement or get vitamin D *preventatively* so that our levels would *already be sufficient* in case we encountered SARS-CoV-2. A study published in the *European Journal of Clinical Nutrition* noted: "*Recent negative interventional trials may be biased by substantial methodological and study design errors, making it impossible to show the potential contributing role of vitamin D supplementation in a deficient population,*"[298]. What does that mean? Due to poor research design, several studies tend to show no positive health effects from vitamin D supplementation.

I saved the best for last. In a paper, boldly titled "COVID-19 mortality risk correlates inversely with vitamin D3 status, and a mortality rate close to zero could theoretically be achieved at 50 ng/ml 25(OH)D3...", suggests exactly what the title says. Vitamin D status is a very strong predictor of severity and death from COVID-19, and according to the researchers, achieving a blood level of 50 ng/ml of 25(OH) vitamin D could—using computer modeling––dramatically bring down the mortality from COVID-19 to near zero. The authors also write:

"...*humanity could be trapped in an insuperable race between new mutations and new vaccines, with an increasing risk of newly arising mutations becoming resistant to the current vaccines... Mask requirements as well as limitations of public life will likely accompany us for a long time if we are not able to establish additional methods that reduce virus dissemination. Vaccination is an important part in the fight against SARS CoV 2 but... should not be the only focus. One strong pillar in the protection against any type of virus infection is the strength of our immune system [12]. Unfortunately, thus far, this unquestioned basic principle of nature has been more or less neglected by the responsible authorities,"* [299]. Mic drop.

Though it would be ideal to obtain all of our vitamins from food or sunlight, it may not be feasible for many people due to location or food availability. While supplementation of vitamin D may be most convenient, skipping the step of converting cholesterol to vitamin D via sunlight exposure (and not a supplement) may be, at least somewhat, important. In fact, studies have shown a moderate decrease in cholesterol when exposed to the sun but not when given a supplement[300]. In addition, blood pressure seems to be slightly higher, and HDL (the "good" cholesterol) seems to be lower in those who have low sun exposure[301]. However, if the goal is simply to raise vitamin D levels as fast/high as possible, supplementation wins[302].

Now, let's talk about magnesium—*again*. Magnesium deficiencies increase the amounts of cytokines in the body. A quick refresher: an abnormally high presence of cytokines is associated with increased inflammation and severity of COVID-19. Magnesium is also involved in *activating* Vitamin D in the body[303]. Therefore, even if you're taking ample amounts of vitamin D, it may not be fully functional without enough magnesium.

Vitamin K has been shown to have a synergistic effect with vitamin D also[304]. Vitamin K's importance in promoting immune health has also been established. Specifically, thromboembolism—think of a traffic jam in your blood vessels—has been observed in severe cases of COVID-19. In these cases, vitamin K becomes even more important, as it can help with anticoagulation of blood which leads to protection against potentially dangerous blood clots[305]. In addition, vitamin K has been shown to be somewhat protective against lung and blood vessel damage, which can occur downstream of viral infections. Vitamin K can be found mainly in organ meats and leafy greens. As always, check with your doctor, as supplements can interfere with medications.

Finally, vitamin A is another important player. Vitamin A is depleted by UV radiation[306]. Therefore, as you spend more time in the sun, getting enough vitamin A from foods like beef liver and eggs is important. Though you could eat some sweet potatoes and carrots, animal foods are optimal since they contain the active forms of vitamin A, while plant-derived vitamin A must be converted into the active form by your body.

Soak up the Free Radicals

Free radicals are agents which can damage DNA, cell membranes, and wreak havoc on our body if not properly balanced by antioxidants. Consuming antioxidant-rich foods, such as dark chocolate[307], wild caught salmon[308], and berries, may be helpful when it comes to improving skin damage and repairing damage to skin caused by sunlight.

One of the most potent antioxidants known to man does not come from food—we make it ourselves. Melatonin, often known as the sleep hormone, does much more than make you drowsy. In fact, melatonin may specifically protect against UVR-induced skin damage[309]. Therefore, consider short-term melatonin supplementation and/or prioritize sleep before and after sun exposure, especially if you do get a sunburn.

This doesn't give you a free pass to lay in the sun for as long as you want. It's important to respect the power of the sun, both for good and for harm. Depending on your skin type, the amount of skin you have exposed, and the UV index, it may be a good idea to invest in a non-toxic sunscreen, such as zinc oxide, and spread out sun exposure time.

RESOURCES AND FURTHER READING
1. Dr. Alexander Wunsch
2. Dr. Jack Kruse
3. Dr. Joshua Rosenthal
4. Dr. Satchin Panda
5. Estimate your vitamin D levels with the "Dminder" app

CHAPTER 8: TAKE THAT OUT OF YOUR POCKET!

No, 5G does not cause COVID-19. When this unfounded theory first came out, I remember experts in the field of bioelectromagnetics being disappointed and frustrated. That baseless claim would take the focus off of the real, scientific dangers of electromagnetic fields. It would also polarize those who already believed that anyone who worried about cellphones and cell towers were a bunch of tinfoil hat-wearing quacks. In other words, it made people dismiss the *valid* evidence that chronic EMF exposure is harmful.

Until a few years ago, I never considered the fact that humans are, in a sense, electromagnetic. From the beating of a heart to the contraction of a muscle—we are powered by electromagnetism. Centuries ago, the electromagnetic fields (EMFs) naturally produced by animals, plants, sunlight, cosmic radiation, and the earth were some of the only sources of EMFs. These natural EMFs are commonly referred to as *native* EMFs. For millions of years, life evolved constantly exposed to these natural EMFs. The modern world paints a much different picture. Now, we are constantly bombarded by radiation from cellphones, WiFi routers, power lines, and more. These man-made electromagnetic fields—known as non-native EMFs––interfere with our body's hormones, circadian rhythms, and internal antioxidant systems. In fact, chronic exposure to these man-made EMFs is linked to insomnia, heart palpitations, arrhythmia, ringing in the ears, anxiety, cancer, and depression. It's important to be clear that some of these are *associations* and may not be direct causes. As with everything else in this book, EMFs may be *a* cause, and likely not *the* cause. How do we know these effects are truly due to our wireless devices? Aren't they proven to be safe? Let me begin by introducing you to the electromagnetic spectrum.

If you've taken a basic physics class, you're probably familiar with the electromagnetic spectrum (I recommend you look up a visual of the electromagnetic spectrum while reading this section). The electromagnetic spectrum includes microwaves, radio waves, visible light, ultraviolet radiation, X-rays, and beyond. We're usually taught that EMFs with the highest frequencies are the most damaging since they deliver the most energy. While this is true, it wrongly assumes that low-frequency radiation—such as radio-frequency radiation (RF) and microwave radiation from cellphones, cell towers, and WiFi—is 100% safe. This is because RF radiation is categorized as *non-ionizing radiation*.

Electromagnetic radiation is divided into two main groups: ionizing and non-ionizing radiation. Ionizing radiation (IR) is defined as mid-to-high energy radiation which can *directly* causing DNA damage (e.g., X-rays)[310]. Non-ionizing radiation can be thought of as IR's little brother—weaker but mischievous nonetheless. Examples of non-IR include extremely low frequency waves (ELF), Radiofrequency (RF) radiation, and microwaves from wireless devices, cell towers, and power lines.

The idea that RF radiation is too weak to affect tissues is a perfect example of the limited narrow-minded thinking which currently plagues the health sciences. Thousands of studies have shown that wireless, non-Ionizing Radiation does indeed affect our cells and tissues. More shocking is the fact that dangers of RF and microwave radiation are *not* new discoveries. As of 1972, U.S. military studies had already been published regarding the numerous biological effects of these types of radiation[311]. Though everyone is biologically affected by electromagnetic radiation, people who are diagnosed with Electrical/Electromagnetic Hypersensitivity have much more obvious symptoms. In fact, the World Health Organization estimates that about **1-10%** of the general population has Electromagnetic Hypersensitivity[312].

If chronic cellphone radiation is such a problem, why do many government and health officials claim it is safe?

First, EMF safety guidelines are *over 20 years old*. When they were established, they only considered *thermal (heating) effects*. Why is that a problem? In the 1980s and 90s, many scientists, health officials, and researchers made the false assumption that heating caused by RF radiation was the *only possible danger*. We now know that EMFs can significantly affect human tissue and organs, *regardless of heat* produced by wireless radiation. According to Dr. Pall, Professor Emeritus of Biochemistry and Basic Medical Sciences at Washington State University, there are eight major types of deleterious effects of EMFs. These effects occur *irrespective of thermal effects*. This is the theorized mechanism of EMFs: "*Produce excessive intracellular calcium [Ca2+]i and excessive calcium signaling*" [313]. Increased calcium in the cell leads to increased free radical formation, oxidative stress, DNA damage, and inflammation[314].

Conflicts of interest have also created confusion surrounding the effects of EMFs on health. Researchers have found that the source of funding profoundly affects the results of a study. 64% of studies which received public or charity funding found a significant biological effect of mobile phone use. On the other hand, only 33% of studies funded by the telecommunications industry found a significant effect of mobile phone use on human health[315].

Next, the safety limits and guidelines in the United States have not been updated to reflect our current scientific understanding and research. Why? Well, partially because the FCC is known as a captured agency. People formerly involved with the telecommunications industry currently hold positions in the FCC, which I don't need to tell you is an obvious conflict of interest. The telecommunications industry wants to roll out as much technology as possible, while the FCC is meant to create safety standards. Therefore, former telecommunication representatives within the FCC understand that stringent regulations would be a barrier towards that goal. The telecom industry also has too much to lose if they admit to the dangers of EMFs.

Outrage, lawsuits, and monetary loss would inevitably ensue. However, several cities in the U.S., as well as other countries, have put their legislative big boy pants on, passing resolutions to halt 5G, do independent testing, and educate their citizens properly about safe tech use.

Thousands of scientists worldwide, independent from industry, have expressed their concerns about wireless radiation emitted from cell towers, cellphones, and WiFi. The International Agency for Research on Cancer (IARC), part of the World Health Organization (WHO), concluded that EMFs at frequencies 30 KHz to 300 GHz are a Group 2B carcinogen to humans[316]. From the Bioinitiative Report in 2012[317], to the multimillion-dollar National Toxicology Program (NTP) study and beyond, the research continues to pile on, showing clear biological effects from wireless radiation. In fact, the NTP study actually demonstrates a *causal* relationship between chronic wireless radiation exposure and certain cancers in animals[318]. The carcinogenic classification of wireless radiation is currently under review and may be updated to a higher level of carcinogenicity (cancer-causing potential).

As I mentioned earlier, Dr. Martin Pall has compiled a document of the 8 major effects from non-thermal microwave frequency EMFs: disruption of the nervous system and endocrine system, increased oxidative stress as well as single and double strand DNA breaks, increased apoptosis (cell death), decreased male and female fertility, and increased cancer promotion within cells[319].

To summarize, studies have demonstrated that RF EMF exposure is linked to:

- Damage to the immune system via increased oxidative stress, impaired tissue repair, alteration of immune cell morphology, and negative effects on bone marrow and white blood cells[320]
- Demyelination of neurons[321]. Myelin, the fatty layer which surrounds neurons to keep them working optimally, is decreased with exposure to EMFs.
- Tumor promotion[322]
- Altered brain activity[323]
- Damaged brain development, hyperactivity disorders in children, and problems with memory[324]
- Damaged brain cells[325]. Abnormally high death of brain cells is also seen in neurodegenerative diseases such as Alzheimer's disease or Parkinson's disease
- Damage to the Blood Brain Barrier, which makes the brain more susceptible to environmental toxins[326]

If you are anything like I am, you may be ready to ditch all worldly belongings, buy a few goats and chickens, move to the countryside, and live off of the land. For most people, of course, this is unimaginably unrealistic. Technology is, and will continue to be, a major part of everyday life for the foreseeable future. Therefore, we must drive industry to make technology safer, as well as *mitigate* negative effects of wireless radiation, rather than renounce modern society to go live in the forest—however intriguing that might sound.

Again, my purpose in writing this section is not

to scare you into a panic, which, in itself, will worsen your health. Although there are some effects of non-ionizing radiation which are *causal,* several others are still just associations. In addition, these findings are testing prolonged, chronic use of EMFs. Unfortunately, most people are attached to their devices, making chronic EMF exposure something to pay attention to.

Rather than fearmongering, here are some simple steps you can take to reduce and mitigate exposure to wireless radiation.

Magnesium, Melatonin, and Omega 3

After so much mention of magnesium, do you see why it's the number one supplement I take? Magnesium is involved with hundreds of biochemical reactions and is largely absent from the modern diet. How can this mineral specifically be helpful in mitigating the negative effects of wireless radiation? Magnesium is a natural *calcium channel blocker*[327]. Remember back to Dr. Pall's research on the mechanism of action of wireless radiation? EMFs from cellphones, microwaves, and other common devices *increase* calcium concentrations in cells. Therefore, in a world plagued by non-native EMFs, adequate magnesium consumption is critical and may help reduce excessive calcium from rushing into our cells.

Another easy action you can take to reduce RF radiation exposure at night is to turn off WiFi. Why? Sleep is the number one mechanism by which restoration and repair occurs in the body. As I explained in the previous chapter on sunlight, melatonin is one of the most potent antioxidants in the body. In addition to its protective effects against UV radiation, melatonin has been shown to be protective against the negative effects from cellphone radiation[328]. Since wireless radiation is linked to crippled immune health—with increased oxidative stress at the core—turning off the WiFi at night will reduce damage to the body at the most critical time of the day.

Finally, researchers found that, in addition to melatonin, Omega 3 protects against the negative effects of cellphone radiation. Again, wild caught sardines, mackerel, salmon, and anchovies are the ultimate superfoods in this case. They are the lowest in heavy metals and the highest in omega 3s. I personally consume omega 3s solely through food and stay away from fish oil supplements since many times the oils are broken down (oxidized) by the time they get to you.

Away from the Body

The closer a cellphone is to the body, the higher the intensity of wireless radiation—in fact, this relationship is exponential. Now, think about where you put your phone. The most common places are either in your bra or in your pocket. Why is this a problem?

In 2017, a study found a 50–60% decline in sperm count in men from North America, Europe, Australia, and New Zealand from 1973-2011. *In vitro* (cell culture) and *in vivo* animal studies have consistently demonstrated decreased sperm count, decreased sperm motility, and damage to sperm DNA[329]. These and many other studies reveal that wireless radiation exposure plays a role in decreased fertility. For women with no history of cancer, an association between prolonged cellphone use and breast cancer has been shown[330]. Clusters of tumors were shown to be present directly where the phone was in direct contact with the skin. There are plenty of other effects linked to prolonged cellphone radiation, including effects on growth, pubertal development, pregnancy, and more[331, 332].

The safety tests conducted by U.S. regulatory agencies are not only more than 20 years outdated, they also *do not test a phone as it is really used*. Phones are tested for safety at a distance, rather than in close proximity to the body (how they're *actually* used). Therefore, they easily pass the safety standards—which we know are already inadequate.

That being said, there is one simple step you can take to reduce the negative effects of wireless radiation. First, keep the phone away from the body. If this is not possible, turn it off or put it in airplane mode when it is near your body. Next, use speakerphone or wired earbuds when making a phone call—refrain from putting a cellphone next to the head as much as possible.

Grounding/Earthing

If you're a skeptic at heart, this will probably sound a bit woo-woo, but stay with me. The practice of grounding/earthing refers to making direct contact with the ground, or even swimming in an ocean or lake. A review article published in the *Journal of Inflammation Research* summarized some of the potential benefits of earthing: improved wound healing (after daily 30-minute grounding sessions), enhanced sleep quality, and decreased inflammation[333].

A randomized controlled trial found that four weeks of grounding led to improvements in mood, fatigue, and physical pain[334]. A clinical trial discussed another fascinating finding: two hours of grounding led to decreased *blood viscosity*[335]. A high blood viscosity would mean your blood is very thick, which impairs blood flow. In fact, high blood viscosity is associated with an increased risk of heart disease[336]. It's also associated with... you guessed it—COVID-19 severity. Higher blood viscosity during COVID-19 infection leads to more blood clotting, which could block blood flow to the lungs (pulmonary embolism) and/or lead to heart failure[337]. I'd love to see studies of COVID-19 patients using grounding mats to see if this effect is truly significant enough to make a difference.

If you believe this to be BS, that's ok. But I urge you to try it out for yourself—it literally can't hurt. And don't just do it once—give it a real chance. Grounding is an under-researched field of study, so the only *real* way to know is to experiment for yourself.

Use Ethernet

Making the switch from wireless connection to wired connection (ethernet) can seem like an unnecessary bother to the average, unaware person. However, if you're still reading, you are no such person. Using a wired connection will radically reduce your exposure to wireless radiation. This is especially important if your health is not optimal, your job requires constant cellphone/computer usage, and if you do not engage in self-care habits in order to mitigate the harmful effects of chronic EMF radiation.

Measure Radiation in Your Home

Measuring the radiation in your home using an RF meter is the best way to determine which rooms most expose you to wireless radiation. After measuring, you can then decide what to do: move to another room in the house, change the location of the WiFi router, turn off power to the house at night, use EMF-proof fabric, EMF-proof paint and so on. To get a professional evaluation of your home, consider hiring a building biologist.

Take Action Locally

No amount of healthy superfoods and supplements will protect us if we are chronically exposed to an unhealthy environment. 5G, which is currently an untested technology, is being rolled out in backyards, feet from people's front doors, in playgrounds, and schools. Again, if you are healthy, eating right, sleeping well, and exercising, you are less likely to be affected—at least, with short term exposure. But in children and developing adolescents, exposure to something which may have permanent effects on the nervous system and endocrine system is not something to take lightly.

Take action locally by visiting the Environmental Health Trust at https://ehtrust.org/take-action-on-5g-and-cell-phone-radiation/.

RESOURCES
1. Environmental Health Trust
2. Physicians for Safe Technology
3. Dr. Devra Davis
4. Dr. Martin Pall
5. Dr. Joel M. Moskowitz
6. Ramazzini Institute
7. Dr. Joshua Rosenthal
8. Dr. Jack Kruse

CHAPTER 9: CAREFUL WITH THE CROSSFIT CRAZE

Movement has been a part of the human experience for as long as we've been human. In fact, it was an absolute necessity. Life or death sprints, prolonged hunts, and long treks in search of food and water encompassed the lives our ancestors used to live. For thousands of years, their survival depended on their ability to *move*.

Although we largely shifted from a hunter-gatherer society to an agricultural one thousands of years ago, that certainly didn't mean we did less physical work. From tilling the soil to carrying heavy equipment, movement was an integral component of life for small family farms. For the most part, movement was either of low-level intensity for hours at a time, or short bursts of strength and power.

We've now reached a point in history where comfort rules. Most people sit for hours at work, sit for hours on the commute to work, and then proceed to lay stagnant in bed. Then, they do it all over again the next day. Needless to say, *what a major disconnect* between the lives our ancestors led for thousands of years and the lives we currently lead! By this point in the book, the consequences of such a lifestyle are quite clear—booming rates of diabetes, heart disease, and an epidemic of obesity.

So, does this mean the more exercise you do the better? Absolutely not. To demonstrate my point, let's take a mental trip to a stereotypical crossfit gym. Banging weights. Deafening music. Grunts of maximum effort. Sweat-painted floors. While I think crossfit can be a very comprehensive exercise, it often seems to come with a culture of overtraining. Although it's clear that a sedentary lifestyle is a problem, the modern culture of *"no pain, no gain",* has created yet another problem. This book has made it clear that modern humans face more man-made everyday stressors than our ancestors. Why is that relevant? Rather than allow adequate rest for adaptation, a strenuous workout routine simply adds to the overall stress load. Though early humans were resilient as hell, the stressors of the modern lifestyle (as evidenced by the previous chapters) have taken a massive toll on the resilience of modern-day humans. Therefore—for most people—a middle ground between totally sedentary and CrossFit maniac is the way to go.

If you are a David Goggins fanatic (and I am too), you might not like to hear this. However, there's a lot of evidence behind the idea that exercise, in certain contexts, can be deleterious to health—specifically, immune health. In fact, several studies have shown that overexercising, specifically endurance exercise, can lead to *immunosuppression*, higher risk of respiratory infections[338], and increased histamine release, as I explained previously. The simplest solutions to this problem would be to listen to your body and cut down on exercise volume, change the types of exercise you do, and/or find ways to recover better (e.g., reduce stress, improve sleep, nutritional protocols).

However, if you're a masochist at heart, there may be some ways around exercise-induced immunosuppression. Consuming carbohydrates during and/or after exercise seem to lower the inflammatory response associated with intense exercise. In addition, omega 3 fats EPA and DHA seem to act similarly and have been shown to specifically reduce IL-6 levels. Finally, getting adequate intake of vitamin D, E, and C may also play a role in decreasing exercise-induced immunosuppression[339].

After searching PubMed for vitamin D's effects on respiratory infections, I found a perfect example of a null result which doesn't actually mean vitamin D doesn't work. In this study, they gave 2,000 IUs per day of vitamin D to swimmers with vitamin D insufficiency (<30 ng/ml), since it is well known that they are at increased risk of upper respiratory infections. They found that after 12 weeks, they only increased vitamin D levels a *measly* average of 5 ng/ml, which, for the most part, *did not even resolve vitamin D insufficiency*[340]!! In other words, the dose and duration of the study were not enough to make their vitamin D levels sufficient. Therefore, it *appears* as if vitamin D is not helpful. However, as I shared in earlier chapters, vitamin D has been shown to be important for health when levels are raised above 40 ng/ml. The problem is that it takes a while.

My point is, exercise can be an added stressor

if your nutrition, sleep, and stress management suck and you embrace the *no pain, no gain* mentality by training Crossfit for 2 hours a day. That being said, incorporating some sort of *movement* every single day is ideal. While excessive sweat, blurry vision, and trembling muscles may make you feel strong and valiant, everyday max effort is masochistic at best. Don't get me wrong, there's a time and place for all out workouts where you go to failure. Unless you are an athlete, a proper workout regimen should leave you feeling energized rather than always depleted.

An intelligent exercise routine can: boost brain health[341], improve cardiovascular fitness, reduce the risk of infections and increase the efficacy of vaccines[342], increase muscle strength, reduce blood sugar, and decrease resting heart rate[343]. What about COVID-19? A study which analyzed 76,395 individuals found: "***The active group** (500–<1000 MET min/week) was found to have **22% lower risk of COVID-19 infection** (aRR (model 2) 0.78; 95% CI 0.66 to 0.92), **38% lower risk of severe COVID-19** (aRR (model 2) 0.62; 95% CI 0.43 to 0.90) and **83% lower risk of COVID-19-related death**,*"[344]. Keep in mind, this study *only* looked at exercise! With exercise *alone*, this group of over 76,000 adults had an 83% lower risk of COVID-19-related death. Imagine if they were also doing some of the other things I've mentioned throughout this book. Another study published in the journal *Mayo Clinic Proceedings* found an inverse relationship between maximal exercise capacity and the risk of complications from COVID-19. Basically, the more intense exercise you were able to sustain—to a certain point—the lower your risk of being hospitalized with COVID-19[345].

Choosing the least stressful days of your week

to do high intensity interval training, sprints, and explosive exercises would make sense. The rest of the days could consist of lower-stress aerobic exercises, lifting weights, walking, jogging, biking, and yoga. Whatever you *like* and can realistically *stick to* should make up the foundation of your workouts. From what I've learned, it seems that building and maintaining muscle is one of the most important things you can do for your health—not just for the aesthetic benefits (although that's a nice plus). Building muscle is important for preventing injuries, keeping your blood sugar in a healthy range, and keeping insulin levels in check. Therefore, I strongly believe that a strength-focused workout regimen is one of the smartest things you can do for your health. Though blanket statements don't come often in this book, I think virtually everyone would benefit from lifting heavy weights a few times a week, while incorporating other types of movement the remaining days of the week.

Before I end this chapter, I want to get *really* clear on what overexercising means—the last thing I want to do is deter someone with good intentions from exercising. Immunosuppression can occur when one has a *training regimen similar to that of an athlete*, and is *not* likely with acute bursts of intensity followed by adequate rest (i.e., a non-athlete's exercise regimen). If you're just a dude or dudette trying to get stronger by lifting 2 or 3 times a week and going on a light jog the remaining days of the week, you will probably be fine.

Everyone reacts differently. Learn to listen to your body as you experiment with movement and exercise regimens. Are you feeling brain fog? Fatigue? Extreme muscle soreness? Inability to recover? Are you making the infamous pain face too often? How is your digestion? If you are data-driven, measuring heart rate during workouts, heart rate variability (HRV) between workouts, and sleep quality and quantity are all great ways to hone in on the "just right" exercise intensities for *your* lifestyle.

All in all, a ripped, Greek god-like physique does *not* necessarily guarantee perfect health—specifically in terms of immunity.

NOW WHAT?

People are as divided as ever before—about everything, not just COVID-19. Now that the vaccines are out and new variants are emerging, the unvaccinated are blaming the vaccinated, while the vaccinated are blaming the unvaccinated. To the "anti-vax" crowd, "pro vax" people are brainwashed sheeple who don't "think critically". To the "pro-vax" crowd, "anti-vaxers" are dangerous, uneducated conspiracy nut jobs who should be silenced at all costs. There are always people on the extremes. The problem is that the news and social media make it seem like those crazy liberals or those fanatic conservatives are *everywhere*. But they aren't. So, when are we going to realize that neither side is totally correct, yet both can give us parts of the truth? When are we going to realize that the vast majority of us are *pro-human*?

If this past year showed us anything it's that few of the scientists, politicians, and health professionals which made the headlines approached the pandemic in a level-headed, unbiased way. If that would have occurred, maybe we would understand the importance and relevance of our evolutionary history. For the past few centuries, modern humans have done an outstanding job of alienating ourselves from nature. By building a literal wall—actually four of them— between ourselves and nature, we have shifted from a life *enriched* with biodiversity, including viruses, to a sterile indoor lifestyle plagued by nutrient-poor food, chronic stress, artificial light, and electromagnetic fields. As the modern stressors pile on exponentially, widespread disease, accelerated aging, and crippled immune health are the obvious consequences.

If all sides of the story were discussed, more people would understand that modern medicine is incredible *acutely* but has severe limitations in treating and preventing chronic disease. Rather than denouncing modern medicine, however, we should enjoy its benefits *and* incorporate ancestral habits learned from populations like the Hadza. Research has shown us their astonishing metabolic, immune, and cardiovascular health, as well as their remarkable life spans and health spans—which rival, and often surpass, those of industrialized nations[346]. The Hadza's high gut microbial diversity and richness, high vitamin D status, physical fitness, metabolic health, and sense of community all contribute to a strong immune system[347]. Sadly, much of the modern medical system myopically focuses on: genetics rather than epigenetics; drugs over lifestyle; symptom management rather than root cause solutions; reductionism rather than holism. *Abusing* this approach has increased lifespan at the expense of healthspan. In other words, a lack of emphasis on healthy lifestyle habits has simply prolonged a low quality of life.

The pandemic has also made it clear that

there's more to blame for our problems than a virus. For example, the link between air pollution and COVID-19 severity is pronounced, but it has received minimal reporting. It is well known that increases in fine particulate matter ($PM_{2.5}$)—which refers to a certain particle size of dirt, metals, and chemicals floating in the air—creates inflammation in the lungs, weakens the immune system and is linked to many co-morbidities. In fact, there are numerous studies which demonstrate that blood clotting and thrombosis—conditions promoted by air pollution—can lead to multi-organ failure which is seen in some patients with severe COVID-19[348]. In addition, researchers found: "...*an increase of only 1 μg/m3 in long-term average $PM_{2.5}$ is associated with a statistically significant 8% increase in the COVID-19 death rate*,"[349]. Other researchers found "...*an increase of 1 μg/m3 in the long-term average $PM_{2.5}$ is associated with a statistically significant 11% (95% CI, 6 to 17%) increase in the county's COVID-19 mortality rate*," [350]. In other words, a relatively *small* decrease in air quality results in a relatively *large* increase in death rate. New York city, one of the cities which was most affected by COVID-19, has one of the highest $PM_{2.5}$ levels nationwide[351]. There is now preliminary evidence that SARS-CoV-2 can hitch a ride on this particulate matter[352]. Otherwise stated, these studies suggest that air pollution not only makes one more likely to develop chronic diseases (indirectly increasing likelihood of poor COVID-19 outcomes), but it also may *directly* facilitate viral particles getting into our lungs. This research adds to the whole point of this book—that the *root cause* of severe disease seen in COVID-19 patients is *not* merely a virus, but rather complications arising from a combination of lifestyle and environmental factors.

Unfortunately, our public health authorities didn't mention any of this. They waited almost a full year into the pandemic to even *mention* the importance of diet and lifestyle—and when they did, they brushed over it in a sentence or two with something along the lines of: "*Yea, I wouldn't mind taking some vitamin D or zinc*". If the importance of lifestyle was emphasized at the start of the pandemic, *millions* of people's lives could have been changed and thousands saved. In fact, it is now estimated that around 575,000 lives could have been prevented merely through *diet and exercise* in the United States alone[353]. If our response to COVID-19 was truly about health—as most politicians claimed—the importance of nutrition, air pollution, sunlight and vitamin D, metabolic health, and exercise would have been shouted from the rooftops. If this was truly about health, not only would those 575,000 people still be with their families, but they would also be experiencing a dramatically higher quality of life. If this was truly about health, we would have been mandated to stop driving our cars, eat whole foods, exercise, walk outside with your shoes off, and meditate like our lives depended on it—because they do.

Basically, we're killing ourselves. Only ~6% of people who died with COVID-19 had no other health conditions[354]. Again, that doesn't mean they were actually healthy, as per the W.H.O. definition of health. The fact is, we aren't truly fighting against a virus—we're fighting against ourselves. Here's how:

- The *millions of tons* of toxic pesticides sprayed into the air, water, and soil yearly
- The chronic exposure to endocrine-disrupting

chemicals which I didn't even get a chance to discuss in this book. For more information on that topic, I recommend checking out Dr. Aly Cohen's book: "Non-Toxic: Guide to Living Healthy in a Chemical World"

- Monocrop agriculture which releases carbon dioxide into the air, destroys ecosystems, and leads to nutrient-poor food[355]
- Chronically over or under-exercising
- The toxic concentrations of air pollution
- Our apparent inability to have a dialogue with someone who has a different opinion
- The unsustainable, high-stress lifestyles of the modern world
- The exponential increase in wireless radiation
- Corrupt scientific research
- The modern healthcare system, which has no focus on educating people to lead healthier lives
- The lack of gratitude, love, and human connection

Trust me, I understand how it sounds. We've been locked away from our friends, faced difficult financial situations, seen friends and family die, and felt the weight of depression and anxiety on our shoulders. The last thing you probably want to hear is that we—all of us humans—are largely responsible for so much destruction. The massive weight of this realization is enough to make you want to bury your head in the sand permanently. But there's a bright side. If we all individually and collectively decide to take this massive burden of responsibility, I choose to believe that *we can do something to change it.*

Our efforts and dollars should be invested in rebuilding a world fit for life, rather than funding the toxic lifestyles we currently lead.

As depressing as it may sound, if we continue on our current destructive path, we may not be here for much longer. We're coming up on the Sixth Major Extinction event, with species going extinct at a faster rate than ever before—largely attributable to human actions[356]. It's estimated that as many as 100,000 species are going extinct every year[357]. Species are dying out before we even get the chance to discover and name them. At our current rate, we only have a few more decades of life left before the majority of life on Earth is *wiped out*. I'd like to believe that we can change that fate. Here are a few steps in the right direction.

Invest in regenerative agriculture and buy local

Monocrop agriculture is the practice of growing gigantic quantities of single crops in enormous fields. Think of a gray, lifeless field of wheat, soy, or corn. This is probably where your veggie burger is coming from.

At the moment, eccentric multibillionaires are looking to create an expensive technology that will sequester carbon from the air. In my humble opinion? We already have *one* possible solution. A large proportion of carbon is taken up into healthy soils[358]. Spoiler alert—healthy soils are not found in monocrop agriculture. This is part of my problem with the vegan movement. Although I understand the allure and think that the intentions are honorable, I think most vegan arguments are out of touch with reality. I see vegan influencers eating processed, plant-based junk food, deluding themselves into thinking they are saving the planet or nourishing their bodies by stuffing themselves with fake burgers which have a paragraph of ingredients—each of which come from either monocrop agriculture or a food lab.

Seriously? We aren't going to save the planet by simply foregoing all animal products. I believe that we *will* make a positive environmental impact by buying local food (plants and animals) from farmers who run regenerative farms—because what does a regenerative farm entail? Both plants *and* animals. Animals fertilize the soil, the grass feeds them, and the results are nutrient dense animal and plant foods. From my understanding, regenerative agriculture is a way to mimic real ecosystems, while commercial agriculture *destroys* ecosystems and displaces animals. Millions of small animals—birds, insects, and rodents—must be killed every year in order to protect giant monocrop fields. So, the next time your vegan friend rants to you about how he/she is saving the earth by eating a soy-isolate burger—imported from thousands of miles away on a fossil-fuel guzzling jet—realize that he/she is probably killing more life and destroying the earth much more than your grass-fed steak (not to mention, you're getting much better nutrition). Obviously, not every vegan fits the stereotype I've discussed above. There are different reasons for wanting to go on different diets. Someone's dietary preferences are not my business. What does concern me is when we start to delude ourselves into believing something is *always* healthy in *all* contexts for *all* people simply because of our emotions. As always, the truth seems to be more complex.

In order to reduce the prevalence of pesticides,

improve soil health, grow nutrient-rich food, and sequester carbon into soils, commercial farming must go.

I also recommend growing some of your own food. If every person in your neighborhood grew just 5% of their own food in their backyard, think of the tremendous impact that would have—less waste, more money saved, and more fresh food. Once you decide to grow *and* cook your own food, you know exactly what's in it—and more importantly, what's *not* in it.

If you want to learn more about agriculture, I recommend getting involved with Farmer's Footprint, an organization rebuilding and restoring biodiversity in soils. Learn about agriculture, soil health, and donate at https://farmersfootprint.us/donate/.

Visit www.localharvest.org to find a farmer's market near you.

Halt 5G

At the moment, this untested technology is being rolled out a few feet from homes, in backyards, on playgrounds, and on top of schools. Visit https://ehtrust.org/take-action-on-5g-and-cell-phone-radiation/ to learn more about taking action in your city, the negative effects of wireless radiation, and how you can protect yourself and your family.

Getting Healthy: Easier Said than Done

While much of what I cover in this book is free, such as sunlight, sleep, meditation and breathwork, I understand that: one, it can be very hard to practically implement these things into a lifestyle; and two, you probably have many more questions. That's why I believe in health coaching—so much so that I got certified as one. Although most people can get dramatically healthier doing the simple, free habits I've mentioned in this book, many people can benefit from working with someone who can help them create long term lifestyle change, whether that be a personal trainer, dietitian, and/or a health coach.

Understanding What it Means to be Human

Although I don't believe all humans are always nice and cooperative, I do believe in our potential to deeply connect with one another. Why? Let's go back to the time when Neanderthals were still walking around the earth. Contrary to popular belief, they were not slow, dumb, and oafish. On the contrary, they were stronger, had better vision, and had larger brains than us, the nimble *homo sapiens*. So, how could we possibly outlive them? Part of the answer lies in our ability to coexist, share ideas, innovate, and pass down knowledge from generation to generation[359]. While we do most of this in the modern world, we've become quite *impersonal*. Thanks to modern technology, we can now travel to the opposite side of the globe in less than a day and meet more people than we could ever form meaningful relationships with. Although I'm grateful for these sociological and technological advances, they have largely made people somewhat *disposable*. We no longer have a tribe that we are born into and with which we *must* face war, famine, and death. We no longer have a tribe to which we *must* be loyal. We no longer have a tribe with which we spend most of our lives, deepening our relationships with each tragedy, successful hunt, and sacred ritual. The modern world is instead characterized by angry tweets, straw man arguments, and personal attacks.

We have so many intelligent humans, but lately, that hasn't mattered much. Despite our intelligence, the U.S. and many other countries have come to a tipping point of polarization. When we look at the "opposing side", we assume the worst because that's what the news tells us to do. Caught up in the busyness of life, many of us unconsciously accept this fate. As a result, little has been accomplished—except for breeding hatred and ignoring what really matters.

***

I've often wondered if, after reading this book, some people will think that I'm advocating for all of us humans to hold hands and sing "Kumbaya" in pitch-perfect harmony. The short answer is: no. The slightly longer answer has to do with how I pulled myself out of that dark place several years ago. I told you at the beginning that it began with friends and family—without them, none of what I'm about to tell you would have been possible. From that point on, I tried to fix myself, which is not something I recommend or advocate for. Due to a combination of fear, shame, guilt, and pride, I chose to not ask for help. Except for two people, no one knew what was going through my head—and even they didn't know it all. Thankfully, the internet allowed me to access more information than I could ever need. In my search for some sort of escape from the relentless storm cloud over my head, I stumbled across a video in which Dr. Gabor Mate spoke about addiction.

"*Addiction?*" I thought to myself. "*How does that have anything to do with me?*" Exhausted and without motivation to do anything but passively learn, I clicked on the video. We often think of drug abuse when we hear the word "addiction". Fortunately, that's not why

I found the video relevant. As I watched, it became clear to me that addiction could be applied to certain behaviors, thoughts, and even feelings. Although there's much more to Dr. Mate's work than what I'm about to tell you, the main takeaway for me was simple, but immensely powerful: compassion. Dr. Mate spoke about losing, or suppressing, parts of yourself as an adaptation to rough times during childhood, leading to some sort of addiction. This addiction/behavior was an attempt to find joy and pleasure. Again, addiction (at least, how it's defined here) is not limited to drug abuse. It could be people-pleasing, exercise addiction, workaholism, perfectionism, etc. In response to this addiction, Dr. Mate advocated for something he calls "compassionate inquiry". Instead of asking yourself, *"WHY do you act this way, you idiot?!"* Dr. Mate calls for an approach which *truly* seeks to understand why you act the way you do. Without compassion, I would have never moved forward. I would have never understood why I arrived at such a dark place so early in my life. I would have never understood why I no longer felt any happiness or motivation. Thanks to Dr. Mate's work, I realized that I rarely had any compassion for myself— even when I recognized that I fit the exact definition of a depressed individual. On the contrary, I *despised* myself for it.

"You live a life most people dream of. You have access to the best quality food, a bed to sleep on every night, clean clothes. What the hell do you have to be depressed about? How pathetic." Yikes. But that's exactly what my inner dialogue was like. As you can imagine, this wasn't very helpful. In fact, it was very much like jamming your thumb into a bleeding wound—it seems like it *could* stop the bleeding, but it really just infects the lesion and makes

it hurt more than it should. From that point on, I began to compassionately inquire why I acted and felt the way I did—and I started to make some real progress. But compassion on its own wasn't enough.

A month or so into the pandemic, I came across an online self-development course which was being offered for free. I enrolled. Unlike most online courses which are total scams, the course material deeply resonated with me. The first few modules asked me to determine my "deepest commitments". Deepest commitments? Basically, they were asking me to reach inside and find out what I valued. After struggling for a bit, I then came up with an interesting question for myself: *"What things would I value if I loved living life?"*. After much contemplation, I ultimately decided on a few: truth, love, and happiness. Merely identifying these values didn't cause me to reach enlightenment, make my third eye explode with light, nor did it allow me to transcend my finite self. Nope. Now it was time for the *real work* to begin. Every single night before bed, I would ask myself: *"What does love, happiness, and truth **feel** like?"* And every single day, *all day* I would relentlessly ask myself if I was embodying those values. If not, it was back to the drawing board—why was I not doing so? Every morning I would wake up and imagine what it would feel like to embody those values. The first few months were the worst—I felt as fake as a vegan burger. But slowly, I began to genuinely *feel* those feelings and act accordingly. Long story short— it has changed everything. And it all started with consciously and ruthlessly *changing my emotional state*— no matter where I was or what I was doing. But if I gave it an honest shot and didn't succeed, I would give myself permission to end my life. Whenever I was on the verge of quitting, I would force myself to imagine my mother's face turn from ghastly pale to uncontrollable sobbing if I went through with it. I'd imagine my father's grief due to a loss so painful that no amount of time would *ever* heal it. I knew the question, *"What could I have done?"* would fill their hearts with immeasurable guilt and unimaginable pain. It would follow them until their very own deathbeds. I knew *I'd* be dead, so I wouldn't have to deal with their pain. But strangely, I couldn't fathom being the cause of so much suffering. So, no matter how fake I felt and no matter how much of a failure I deemed myself to be, I kept going.

This whole process was happening concurrently with the writing of this book. Interestingly, with each sentence, paragraph, and page I wrote, I found myself becoming a different person, staring at my words from an entirely new perspective. Every time I opened the document, I'd find words which seemed alien to me, leading me to delete entire pages at a time. Did I really write that? It was as if the pages I had spent hours crafting were written by a complete stranger. At first, I was often disappointed and angry at myself for having written pure rhetoric I had heard on podcasts. Looking back to when I began the book, I now realize that I had not *earned* the knowledge I was espousing—at that point, it was just *information*. With each writing session, however, I became increasingly critical of myself and the words I was writing, combing through primary sources to stay true to my purpose. With each writing session, *information* transformed into *knowledge,* a small portion of which has transformed into *wisdom*. With each writing session, I learned more about the inner workings of my mind, motivations, and actions. I began to be more genuinely compassionate, acknowledge what I don't know, and ruthlessly question everything in search of the truth—even if it made me uncomfortable. If not for compassion, this process would have been *impossible*—I simply would have torn myself down until I deleted this document (and I almost did).

Simply put, I can't think of anything the world needs more than compassion and an open mind. But not just compassion for compassion's sake! We need compassion in order to *inquire*. We need compassion in order to *change*. Without it, we can't open ourselves up to new ideas which challenge our own. In other words, *we're stuck*. If you look around, people are indeed stuck, latching on to catchy headlines they've read on the news, rather than investigating a subject deeply. I've realized that most people cannot debate with logic why they so rabidly believe what they believe, but that hasn't stopped them from shunning family and friends from Thanksgiving or Christmas; that hasn't stopped them from hurling vitriol at people they love; it certainly hasn't stopped them from assuming the worst about anyone who has a different opinion than them.

Instead of acknowledging what we don't know and recognizing our shared humanity, we've chosen to treat people on the "opposite side" as if they're the dumb ones. *"How the hell could they possibly believe that?! How pathetic."* Like my own inner dialogue, this isn't actually a question—it's an attack. Instead of compassionately inquiring, people don't actually seem interested in the answer—because they think they already have it. They seem more interested in deluding themselves into believing they are correct rather than finding the truth, just as I did when I began writing this book. But if we want to find solutions to complex problems, we *must* lead with compassion. It allowed me to forgive myself and allowed me to work towards a solution. It kept me from adding more weight to the ever-increasing burden of life. It kept me alive.

As we reach the end of the book, I must admit something which few health gurus would ever want to openly admit about their carefully crafted book. As the years roll on, the science about nutrition, lifestyle, sleep, COVID-19, and beyond, will have evolved. As time passes, some—if not, *many*—parts of my book will slowly become outdated. That's great! I realize now that *what* I learned is nowhere near as important as *how* I learned it. I've learned to think critically, let go of (some) biases, and find new ways of interacting with the world so that I can maximize my short time alive. I hope to continue on that path, and I hope I inspired you to do the same.

I also want to thank you: for having an open mind; for existing (without you, I would have had no reason to be as rigorous as I was in writing this book); for believing that that a book written by a 21-year-old dude would be worth your time and money. I sincerely hope it was.

I started writing this book on an unstable foundation. I had recently decided to continue living—not because I wanted to, but because I owed it to the people who loved me. I *needed* to find a way to live. For them.

Out of desperation, I began this book, *preaching* that we should return to human—even though I felt faker than Monopoly money and had no real idea what "return to human" even meant. As I write these final words, I realize that this book ended up being just what *I* *needed* to begin learning the true meaning of that catchy title.

ABOUT THE AUTHOR

At the time of writing this, my brain is still developing. I'm currently 21 years old, studying neuroscience in college, while studying nutrition, metabolism, longevity, and physiology in my spare time. I have a strong disdain for half-truths and hold a burning desire to figure out the confusing world we live in.

I realize many of my points are probably controversial. I welcome honest discussion and I am open to changing my mind, but I will not tolerate close-minded, fruitless, or insult-driven arguments.

I am available for individual and small group health/nutrition coaching sessions, working with people to transform their health using a personalized approach to behavior change. My website is livedamnwell.com where you can find articles and podcast episodes about mindset, nutrition, fitness, and anything related to health and wellness. If you have feedback, questions, or would like to schedule a coaching session, go to livedamnwell.com to contact me.

REFERENCES

[1] CONSTITUTION OF THE WORLD HEALTH ORGANIZATION. *Basic Documents*, Forty-fifth edition, Supplement, October 2006

[2] Smits SA, Leach J, Sonnenburg ED, et al. Seasonal cycling in the gut microbiome of the Hadza hunter-gatherers of Tanzania. *Science*. 2017;357(6353):802-806. doi:10.1126/science.aan4834

[3] Marlowe FW, Berbesque JC. Tubers as fallback foods and their impact on Hadza hunter-gatherers. Am J Phys Anthropol. 2009;140(4):751-758. doi:10.1002/ajpa.21040

[4] Gurven, M., & Kaplan, H. (2007). Longevity Among Hunter- Gatherers: A Cross-Cultural Examination. Population and Development Review, 33(2), 321–365. doi:10.1111/j.1728-4457.2007.00171.x

[5] Pontzer H, Wood BM, Raichlen DA. Hunter-gatherers as models in public health. *Obes Rev*. 2018;19 Suppl 1:24-35. doi:10.1111/obr.12785

[6] Bethell CD, Kogan MD, Strickland BB, Schor EL, Robertson J, Newacheck PW. A national and state profile of leading health problems and health care quality for US children: key insurance disparities and across-state variations. Acad Pediatr. 2011;11(3 Suppl):S22-S33. doi:10.1016/j.acap.2010.08.011

[7] CDC. *National Center for Chronic Disease Prevention and Health Promotion (NCCDPHP*

[8] NCHS Data Brief No. 360, February 2020. Prevalence of Obesity and Severe Obesity Among Adults: United States, 2017–2018

[9] Centers for Disease Control and Prevention. *National Diabetes Statistics Report 2020 Estimates of Diabetes and its Burden on the United States*

[10] Moore JX, Chaudhary N, Akinyemiju T. Metabolic Syndrome Prevalence by Race/Ethnicity and Sex in the United States, National Health and Nutrition Examination Survey, 1988–2012. Prev Chronic Dis 2017;14:160287.

DOI: http://dx.doi.org/10.5888/pcd14.160287
[11] Dinse GE, Parks CG, Weinberg CR, et al. Increasing Prevalence of Antinuclear Antibodies in the United States. *Arthritis Rheumatol.* 2020;72(6):1026-1035. doi:10.1002/art.41214
[12] CDC Provisional Death Counts for Coronavirus Disease 2019. Table 3: Conditions contributing to deaths involving coronavirus disease 2019 (COVID-19), by age group, United States. Week ending 2/1/2020 to 8/29/2020.
[13] https://www.franklintempleton.com/investor/tools-and-resources/investor-education/gallup-study
[14] *Research and Development in the Pharmaceutical Industry.* April 2021. Congressional Budget Office. https://www.cbo.gov/publication/57025
[15] NSF, NIH. Federal Funds for R&D. American Association for the Advancement of Science.
[16] Szaszi K. A basic scientist's reflections on research funding. *Can J Kidney Health Dis.* 2015;2:50. Published 2015 Dec 1. doi:10.1186/s40697-015-0087-0

[17] Joynson C, Leyser O. The culture of scientific research. *F1000Res.* 2015;4:66. Published 2015 Mar 13. doi:10.12688/f1000research.6163.1
[18] Ioannidis JP. Why most published research findings are false. *PLoS Med.* 2005;2(8):e124. doi:10.1371/journal.pmed.0020124
[19] Ioannidis JPA. Hundreds of thousands of zombie randomised trials circulate among us. *Anaesthesia.* 2021;76(4):444-447. doi:10.1111/anae.15297
[20] Boughton SL, Wilkinson J, Bero L. When beauty is but skin deep: dealing with problematic studies in systematic reviews. *Cochrane Database Syst Rev.* 2021;6:ED000152. Published 2021 Jun 3. doi:10.1002/14651858.ED000152
[21] Chalmers, I., & Glasziou, P. (2009). Avoidable waste in the production and reporting of research evidence. The Lancet, 374(9683), 86–89. doi:10.1016/s0140-6736(09)60329-9

[22] Scherer RW, Langenberg P, von Elm E. Full publication of results initially presented in abstracts. Cochrane Database Syst Rev 2007; 2: MR000005.
[23] Tallon D, Chard J, Dieppe P. Relation between agendas of the research community and the research consumer. Lancet 2000; 355: 2037–40.
[24] Lexchin J, Bero LA, Djulbegovic B, Clark O. Pharmaceutical industry sponsorship and research outcome and quality: systematic review. *BMJ*. 2003;326(7400):1167-1170. doi:10.1136/bmj.326.7400.1167
[25] Moher D, Pham B, Jones A, et al. Does quality of reports of randomised trials affect estimates of intervention efficacy reported in meta-analyses?. *Lancet*. 1998;352(9128):609-613. doi:10.1016/S0140-6736(98)01085-X
[26] Lilienfeld SO. Psychology's Replication Crisis and the Grant Culture: Righting the Ship. *Perspect Psychol Sci*. 2017;12(4):660-664. doi:10.1177/1745691616687745
[27] Lilienfeld SO. Psychology's Replication Crisis and the Grant Culture: Righting the Ship. *Perspect Psychol Sci*. 2017;12(4):660-664. doi:10.1177/1745691616687745
[28] https://blogs.bmj.com/bmj/2021/07/05/time-to-assume-that-health-research-is-fraudulent-until-proved-otherwise/
[29] National Center for Chronic Disease Prevention and Health Promotion (US) Office on Smoking and Health. The Health Consequences of Smoking—50 Years of Progress: A Report of the Surgeon General. Atlanta (GA): Centers for Disease Control and Prevention (US); 2014. 2, Fifty Years of Change 1964–2014. Available from: https://www.ncbi.nlm.nih.gov/books/NBK294310/
[30] Shehata AA, Schrödl W, Aldin AA, Hafez HM, Krüger M. The effect of glyphosate on potential pathogens and beneficial members of poultry microbiota in vitro. *Curr Microbiol*. 2013;66(4):350-358. doi:10.1007/s00284-012-0277-2

[31] Peillex C, Pelletier M. The impact and toxicity of glyphosate and glyphosate-based herbicides on health and immunity. *J Immunotoxicol.* 2020;17(1):163-174. doi:10.1080/1547691X.2020.1804492

[32] McCully KS. Environmental Pollution, Oxidative Stress and Thioretinaco Ozonide: Effects of Glyphosate, Fluoride and Electromagnetic Fields on Mitochondrial Dysfunction in Carcinogenesis, Atherogenesis and Aging. *Ann Clin Lab Sci.* 2020;50(3):408-411.

[33] Rueda-Ruzafa L, Cruz F, Roman P, Cardona D. Gut microbiota and neurological effects of glyphosate. *Neurotoxicology.* 2019;75:1-8. doi:10.1016/j.neuro.2019.08.006

[34] Caiati C, Pollice P, Favale S, Lepera ME. The Herbicide Glyphosate and Its Apparently Controversial Effect on Human Health: An Updated Clinical Perspective. *Endocr Metab Immune Disord Drug Targets.* 2020;20(4):489-505. doi:10.2174/1871530319666191015191614

[35] McHenry LB. The Monsanto Papers: Poisoning the scientific well. *Int J Risk Saf Med.* 2018;29(3-4):193-205. doi:10.3233/JRS-180028

[36] Samet JM. Expert Review Under Attack: Glyphosate, Talc, and Cancer. Am J Public Health. 2019;109(7):976-978. doi:10.2105/AJPH.2019.305131

[37] Robin Mesnage, Maxime Teixeira, Daniele Mandrioli, Laura Falcioni, Quinten Raymond Ducarmon, Romy Daniëlle Zwittink, Caroline Amiel, Jean-Michel Panoff, Fiorella Belpoggi, Michael N Antoniou. 2019. Shotgun metagenomics and metabolomics reveal glyphosate alters the gut microbiome of Sprague-Dawley rats by inhibiting the shikimate pathway. bioRxiv 870105; doi: https://doi.org/10.1101/870105

[38] Lozano VL, Defarge N, Rocque LM, et al. (2018) Sex-dependent impact of Roundup on the rat gut microbiome. *Toxicol Rep* **5**:96–107 doi: 10.1016/j.toxrep.2017.12.005

[39] Mao Q, Manservisi F, Panzacchi S, et al. (2018) The

Ramazzini Institute 13-week pilot study on glyphosate and Roundup administered at human-equivalent dose to Sprague Dawley rats: effects on the microbiome. Environ Health 17(1):50 doi: 10.1186/s12940-018-0394-x

[40] Nielsen LN, Roager HM, Casas ME, et al. (2018) Glyphosate has limited short-term effects on commensal bacterial community composition in the gut environment due to sufficient aromatic amino acid levels. Environmental Pollution 233:364–376 doi: https://doi.org/10.1016/j.envpol.2017.10.016

[41] Valdes Ana M, Walter Jens, Segal Eran, Spector Tim D. Role of the gut microbiota in nutrition and health BMJ 2018; 361 :k2179

[42] https://www.epa.gov/ingredients-used-pesticide-products/glyphosate

[43] Benbrook, C.M. How did the US EPA and IARC reach diametrically opposed conclusions on the genotoxicity of glyphosate-based herbicides?. *Environ Sci Eur* **31,** 2 (2019). https://doi.org/10.1186/s12302-018-0184-7

[44] Silver MK, Fernandez J, Tang J, et al. Prenatal Exposure to Glyphosate and Its Environmental Degradate, Aminomethylphosphonic Acid (AMPA), and Preterm Birth: A Nested Case-Control Study in the PROTECT Cohort (Puerto Rico). Environ Health Perspect. 2021;129(5):57011. doi:10.1289/EHP7295

[45] Keys A. Seven countries: a multivariate analysis of death and coronary heart disease. London: Harvard University Press, 1980.

[46] Anderson JT, Grande F, Keys A. Hydrogenated fats in the diet and lipids in the serum of man. *J Nutr.* 1961;75(4):388-394. doi:10.1093/jn/75.4.388

[47] Ramsden Christopher E, Zamora Daisy, Majchrzak-Hong Sharon, Faurot Keturah R, Broste Steven K, Frantz Robert P et al. Re-evaluation of the traditional diet-heart hypothesis: analysis of recovered data from Minnesota Coronary Experiment (1968-73) BMJ 2016; 353 :i1246

48 Kearns CE, Schmidt LA, Glantz SA. Sugar Industry and Coronary Heart Disease Research: A Historical Analysis of Internal Industry Documents [published correction appears in JAMA Intern Med. 2016 Nov 1;176(11):1729]. *JAMA Intern Med.* 2016;176(11):1680-1685. doi:10.1001/jamainternmed.2016.5394

49 Malhotra A, Redberg RF, Meier P. Saturated fat does not clog the arteries: coronary heart disease is a chronic inflammatory condition, the risk of which can be effectively reduced from healthy lifestyle interventions. *Br J Sports Med.* 2017;51(15):1111-1112. doi:10.1136/bjsports-2016-097285

50 DiNicolantonio JJ, OKeefe JH. Added sugars drive coronary heart disease via insulin resistance and hyperinsulinaemia: a new paradigm. Open Heart. 2017;4(2):e000729. Published 2017 Nov 29. doi:10.1136/openhrt-2017-000729

51 Kratz M. Dietary cholesterol, atherosclerosis and coronary heart disease. *Handb Exp Pharmacol.* 2005;(170):195-213. doi:10.1007/3-540-27661-0_6

52 Gao S, Zhao D, Wang M, et al. Association Between Circulating Oxidized LDL and Atherosclerotic Cardiovascular Disease: A Meta-analysis of Observational Studies. Can J Cardiol. 2017;33(12):1624-1632. doi:10.1016/j.cjca.2017.07.015

53 https://www.nutritioncoalition.us/news/saturated-fat-limit-not-justified

54 Lee BJ, Lin JS, Lin YC, Lin PT. Effects of L-carnitine supplementation on oxidative stress and antioxidant enzymes activities in patients with coronary artery disease: a randomized, placebo-controlled trial. *Nutr J.* 2014;13:79. Published 2014 Aug 4. doi:10.1186/1475-2891-13-79

55 Topi Hovinen, Liisa Korkalo, Riitta Freese, Essi Skaffari, Pirjo Isohanni, Mikko Niemi, Jaakko Nevalainen, Helena Gylling, Nicola Zamboni, Maijaliisa Erkkola, Anu Suomalainen. Vegan diet in young children remodels metabolism and challenges the statuses of essential

nutrients. *EMBO Molecular Medicine*, 2021;
DOI: 10.15252/emmm.202013492

[56] Šamec D, Urlić B, Salopek-Sondi B. Kale (*Brassica oleracea* var. *acephala*) as a superfood: Review of the scientific evidence behind the statement. *Crit Rev Food Sci Nutr*. 2019;59(15):2411-2422.
doi:10.1080/10408398.2018.1454400

[57] Dolan LC, Matulka RA, Burdock GA. Naturally occurring food toxins. *Toxins (Basel)*. 2010;2(9):2289-2332.
doi:10.3390/toxins2092289

[58] Sandip T. Gaikwad, Pradnya Gaikwad, and Vikas Saxena. 2017. Principles of Fasting in Ayurveda.
International Journal of Science, Environment and Technology. Vol. 6, No 1, 787-792.

[59] Yang CS, Chen G, Wu Q. Recent scientific studies of a traditional chinese medicine, tea, on prevention of chronic diseases. J Tradit Complement Med. 2014;4(1):17-23.
doi:10.4103/2225-4110.124326

[60] Saini R. Coenzyme Q10: The essential nutrient. *J Pharm Bioallied Sci*. 2011;3(3):466-467. doi:10.4103/0975-7406.84471

[61] Ruud H J terter Meulen RH. The ethical basis of the precautionary principle in health care decision making. *Toxicol Appl Pharmacol*. 2005;207(2 Suppl):663-667. doi:10.1016/j.taap.2004.11.032

[62] Smith R. Thoughts for new medical students at a new medical school. *BMJ*. 2003;327(7429):1430-1433. doi:10.1136/bmj.327.7429.1430

[63] Tai-Seale M, Olson CW, Li J, et al. Electronic Health Record Logs Indicate That Physicians Split Time Evenly Between Seeing Patients And Desktop Medicine. *Health Aff (Millwood)*. 2017;36(4):655-662.
doi:10.1377/hlthaff.2016.0811

[64] Alper BS, Hand JA, Elliott SG, et al. How much effort is needed to keep up with the literature relevant for primary care?. *J Med Libr Assoc*. 2004;92(4):429-437.

[65] https://www.gov.uk/government/news/jcvi-issues-

advice-on-covid-19-vaccination-of-children-and-young-people
66 Willett WC, Stampfer MJ. Rebuilding the food pyramid. *Sci Am*. 2003;288(1):64-71. doi:10.1038/scientificamerican0103-64
67 Lee, W.S., Wheatley, A.K., Kent, S.J. *et al*. Antibody-dependent enhancement and SARS-CoV-2 vaccines and therapies. *Nat Microbiol* **5,** 1185–1191 (2020). https://doi.org/10.1038/s41564-020-00789-5
68 Cardozo T, Veazey R. Informed consent disclosure to vaccine trial subjects of risk of COVID-19 vaccines worsening clinical disease. Int J Clin Pract. 2021;75(3):e13795. doi:10.1111/ijcp.13795
69 Yahi N, Chahinian H, Fantini J. Infection-enhancing anti-SARS-CoV-2 antibodies recognize both the original Wuhan/D614G strain and Delta variants. A potential risk for mass vaccination? [published online ahead of print, 2021 Aug 9]. J Infect. 2021;S0163-4453(21)00392-3. doi:10.1016/j.jinf.2021.08.010
70 Kostoff RN, Briggs MB, Porter AL, Spandidos DA, Tsatsakis A. [Comment] COVID-19 vaccine safety. *Int J Mol Med*. 2020;46(5):1599-1602. doi:10.3892/ijmm.2020.4733
71 Kipshidze N, Kipshidze N, Fried M. COVID-19 Vaccines: Special Considerations for the Obese Population. Obes Surg. 2021;31(8):3854-3856. doi:10.1007/s11695-021-05404-y
72
Sivan Gazit, Roei Shlezinger, Galit Perez, Roni Lotan, Asaf Peretz, Amir Ben-Tov, Dani Cohen, Khitam Muhsen, Gabriel Chodick, Tal Patalon. Comparing SARS-CoV-2 natural immunity to vaccine-induced immunity: reinfections versus breakthrough infections.
medRxiv 2021.08.24.21262415; doi: https://doi.org/10.1101/2021.08.24.21262415
73 Lumley SF, Rodger G, Constantinides B, et al. An

observational cohort study on the incidence of SARS-CoV-2 infection and B.1.1.7 variant infection in healthcare workers by antibody and vaccination status [published online ahead of print, 2021 Jul 3]. Clin Infect Dis. 2021;ciab608. doi:10.1093/cid/ciab608

[74] Dan JM, Mateus J, Kato Y, et al. Immunological memory to SARS-CoV-2 assessed for up to 8 months after infection. *Science*. 2021;371(6529):eabf4063. doi:10.1126/science.abf4063

[75] Bertoletti A, Le Bert N, Qui M, Tan AT. SARS-CoV-2-specific T cells in infection and vaccination [published online ahead of print, 2021 Sep 1]. Cell Mol Immunol. 2021;1-6. doi:10.1038/s41423-021-00743-3

[76] Wang, Z., Yang, X., Zhong, J. et al. Exposure to SARS-CoV-2 generates T-cell memory in the absence of a detectable viral infection. Nat Commun 12, 1724 (2021). https://doi.org/10.1038/s41467-021-22036-z

[77] Rodda LB, Netland J, Shehata L, et al. Functional SARS-CoV-2-Specific Immune Memory Persists after Mild COVID-19. Cell. 2021;184(1):169-183.e17. doi:10.1016/j.cell.2020.11.029

[78] Cromer, D., Juno, J.A., Khoury, D. *et al.* Prospects for durable immune control of SARS-CoV-2 and prevention of reinfection. *Nat Rev Immunol* **21,** 395–404 (2021). https://doi.org/10.1038/s41577-021-00550-x

[79] Yang Y, Du L. SARS-CoV-2 spike protein: a key target for eliciting persistent neutralizing antibodies. *Signal Transduct Target Ther*. 2021;6(1):95. Published 2021 Feb 26. doi:10.1038/s41392-021-00523-5

[80] Cohen KW, Linderman SL, Moodie Z, et al. Longitudinal analysis shows durable and broad immune memory after SARS-CoV-2 infection with persisting antibody responses and memory B and T cells. Preprint. *medRxiv*. 2021;2021.04.19.21255739. Published 2021 Jun 18. doi:10.1101/2021.04.19.21255739

[81] Jones JM, Stone M, Sulaeman H, et al. Estimated US Infection- and Vaccine-Induced SARS-CoV-2

Seroprevalence Based on Blood Donations, July 2020-May 2021 [published online ahead of print, 2021 Sep 2]. JAMA. 2021;e2115161. doi:10.1001/jama.2021.15161

82 Christie Aschwanden. Five reasons why COVID herd immunity is probably impossible. *Nature* News Feature. 2021. https://www.nature.com/articles/d41586-021-00728-2

83 Vitiello A, Ferrara F, Troiano V, La Porta R. COVID-19 vaccines and decreased transmission of SARS-CoV-2 [published online ahead of print, 2021 Jul 19]. Inflammopharmacology. 2021;1-4. doi:10.1007/s10787-021-00847-2

84 Kasen K. Riemersma, Brittany E. Grogan, Amanda Kita-Yarbro, Peter J. Halfmann, Hannah E. Segaloff, Anna Kocharian, Kelsey R. Florek, Ryan Westergaard, Allen Bateman, Gunnar E. Jeppson, Yoshihiro Kawaoka, David H. O'Connor, Thomas C. Friedrich, Katarina M. Grande. Shedding of Infectious SARS-CoV-2 Despite Vaccination. medRxiv 2021.07.31.21261387; doi: https://doi.org/10.1101/2021.07.31.21261387

85 Kawasuji H, Takegoshi Y, Kaneda M, et al. Transmissibility of COVID-19 depends on the viral load around onset in adult and symptomatic patients. PLoS One. 2020;15(12):e0243597. Published 2020 Dec 9. doi:10.1371/journal.pone.0243597

86 Koen B. Pouwels, Emma Pritchard, Philippa C. Matthews, Nicole Stoesser, David W. Eyre, Karina-Doris Vihta, Thomas House, Jodie Hay, John I Bell, John N Newton, Jeremy Farrar, Derrick Crook, Duncan Cook, Emma Rourke, Ruth Studley, Tim Peto, Ian Diamond, A. Sarah Walker, and the COVID-19 Infection Survey Team. Impact of Delta on viral burden and vaccine effectiveness against new SARS-CoV-2 infections in the UK. Impact of Delta on viral burden and vaccine effectiveness against new SARS-CoV-2 infections in the UK. medRxiv 2021.08.18.21262237; doi: https://doi.org/10.11

01/2021.08.18.21262237

[87] Brown CM, Vostok J, Johnson H, et al. Outbreak of SARS-CoV-2 Infections, Including COVID-19 Vaccine Breakthrough Infections, Associated with Large Public Gatherings - Barnstable County, Massachusetts, July 2021. *MMWR Morb Mortal Wkly Rep*. 2021;70(31):1059-1062. Published 2021 Aug 6. doi:10.15585/mmwr.mm7031e2

[88] Subramanian SV, Kumar A. Increases in COVID-19 are unrelated to levels of vaccination across 68 countries and 2947 counties in the United States [published online ahead of print, 2021 Sep 30]. Eur J Epidemiol. 2021;1-4. doi:10.1007/s10654-021-00808-7

[89] Po Ying Chia, Sean Wei Xiang Ong, Calvin J Chiew, Li Wei Ang, Jean-Marc Chavatte, Tze-Minn Mak, Lin Cui, Shirin Kalimuddin, Wan Ni Chia, Chee Wah Tan, Louis Yi Ann Chai, Seow Yen Tan, Shuwei Zheng, Raymond Tzer Pin Lin, Linfa Wang, Yee-Sin Leo, Vernon J Lee, David Chien Lye, Barnaby Edward Young. Virological and serological kinetics of SARS-CoV-2 Delta variant vaccine-breakthrough infections: a multi-center cohort study. medRxiv 2021.07.28.21261295; doi: https://doi.org/10.11 01/2021.07.28.21261295

[90] Terracina KA, Tan FK. Flare of rheumatoid arthritis after COVID-19 vaccination [published online ahead of print, 2021 Mar 30]. *Lancet Rheumatol*. 2021;10.1016/S2665-9913(21)00108-9. doi:10.1016/S2665-9913(21)00108-9

[91] https://www.cdc.gov/coronavirus/2019-ncov/hcp/planning-scenarios.html#table-1

[92] Seoane B. A scaling approach to estimate the age-dependent COVID-19 infection fatality ratio from incomplete data. PLoS One. 2021;16(2):e0246831. Published 2021 Feb 17. doi:10.1371/journal.pone.0246831

[93] Levin AT, Hanage WP, Owusu-Boaitey N, Cochran KB, Walsh SP, Meyerowitz-Katz G. Assessing the age specificity of infection fatality rates for COVID-19:

systematic review, meta-analysis, and public policy
implications. *Eur J Epidemiol.* 2020;35(12):1123-1138.
doi:10.1007/s10654-020-00698-1

[94] Seoane B. A scaling approach to estimate the age-
dependent COVID-19 infection fatality ratio from
incomplete data. PLoS One. 2021;16(2):e0246831.
Published 2021 Feb 17. doi:10.1371/journal.pone.0246831

[95] O'Driscoll, M., Ribeiro Dos Santos, G., Wang, L. et
al. Age-specific mortality and immunity patterns of SARS-
CoV-2. Nature 590, 140–145
(2021). https://doi.org/10.1038/s41586-020-2918-0

[96] Lopez-Leon S, Wegman-Ostrosky T, Perelman C, et al.
More than 50 Long-term effects of COVID-19: a
systematic review and meta-analysis. Preprint. medRxiv.
2021;2021.01.27.21250617. Published 2021 Jan 30.
doi:10.1101/2021.01.27.21250617

[97] https://www.thennt.com/review-covid-analysis-2020/

[98] Vaccines and Related Biological Products Advisory
Committee Meeting December 10, 2020. FDA Briefing
Document Pfizer-BioNTech COVID-19 Vaccine

[99] https://www.thennt.com/review-covid-analysis-2020/

[100] Olliaro P, Torreele E, Vaillant M. COVID-19 vaccine
efficacy and effectiveness-the elephant (not) in the room
[published online ahead of print, 2021 Apr 20]. *Lancet
Microbe.* 2021;10.1016/S2666-5247(21)00069-0.
doi:10.1016/S2666-5247(21)00069-0

[101] Kostoff RN, Briggs MB, Porter AL, Spandidos DA,
Tsatsakis A. [Comment] COVID-19 vaccine safety. *Int J
Mol Med.* 2020;46(5):1599-1602.
doi:10.3892/ijmm.2020.4733

[102] Santin AD, Scheim DE, McCullough PA, Yagisawa M,
Borody TJ. Ivermectin: a multifaceted drug of Nobel
prize-honoured distinction with indicated efficacy against a
new global scourge, COVID-19. New Microbes New
Infect. 2021;43:100924. Published 2021 Aug 3.
doi:10.1016/j.nmni.2021.100924

[103] DiNicolantonio JJ, Barroso-Aranda J, McCarty MF.

Anti-inflammatory activity of ivermectin in late-stage COVID-19 may reflect activation of systemic glycine receptors. *Open Heart*. 2021;8(1):e001655. doi:10.1136/openhrt-2021-001655

[104] Kory P, Meduri GU, Varon J, Iglesias J, Marik PE. Review of the Emerging Evidence Demonstrating the Efficacy of Ivermectin in the Prophylaxis and Treatment of COVID-19. *Am J Ther*. 2021;28(3):e299-e318. Published 2021 Apr 22. doi:10.1097/MJT.0000000000001377

[105] Bryant A, Lawrie TA, Dowswell T, et al. Ivermectin for Prevention and Treatment of COVID-19 Infection: A Systematic Review, Meta-analysis, and Trial Sequential Analysis to Inform Clinical Guidelines [published online ahead of print, 2021 Jun 17]. *Am J Ther*. 2021;10.1097/MJT.0000000000001402. doi:10.1097/MJT.0000000000001402

[106] Heidary F, Gharebaghi R. Ivermectin: a systematic review from antiviral effects to COVID-19 complementary regimen. *J Antibiot (Tokyo)*. 2020;73(9):593-602. doi:10.1038/s41429-020-0336-z

[107] Roman YM, Burela PA, Pasupuleti V, Piscoya A, Vidal JE, Hernandez AV. Ivermectin for the treatment of COVID-19: A systematic review and meta-analysis of randomized controlled trials [published online ahead of print, 2021 Jun 28]. *Clin Infect Dis*. 2021;ciab591. doi:10.1093/cid/ciab591

[108] Tanveer S, Rowhani-Farid A, Hong K, Jefferson T, Doshi P. Transparency of COVID-19 vaccine trials: decisions without data [published online ahead of print, 2021 Aug 9]. BMJ Evid Based Med. 2021;bmjebm-2021-111735. doi:10.1136/bmjebm-2021-111735

[109] Hodgson SH, Mansatta K, Mallett G, Harris V, Emary KRW, Pollard AJ. What defines an efficacious COVID-19 vaccine? A review of the challenges assessing the clinical efficacy of vaccines against SARS-CoV-2. *Lancet Infect Dis*. 2021;21(2):e26-e35. doi:10.1016/S1473-3099(20)30773-8

[110] Doshi P. Covid-19 vaccines: In the rush for regulatory

approval, do we need more
data? BMJ 2021; 373 :n1244 doi:10.1136/bmj.n1244
[111] Iheanacho CO, Eze UIH, Adida EA. A systematic review of effectiveness of BNT162b2 mRNA and ChAdOx1 adenoviral vector COVID-19 vaccines in the general population. Bull Natl Res Cent. 2021;45(1):150. doi:10.1186/s42269-021-00607-w
[112] https://clinicaltrials.gov/ct2/show/NCT04368728
[113] Kevin J. Hickey. The PREP Act and COVID-19: Limiting Liability for Medical Countermeasures. *Congressional Research Service.* LSB10443.
[114] Wendy C King, Max Rubinstein, Alex Reinhart, Robin J. Mejia. Time trends and factors related to COVID-19 vaccine hesitancy from January-May 2021 among US adults: Findings from a large-scale national survey. medRxiv 2021.07.20.21260795; doi: https://doi.org/10.11 01/2021.07.20.21260795
[115] Arjun Puranik, Patrick J. Lenehan, Eli Silvert, Michiel J.M. Niesen, Juan Corchado-Garcia, John C. O'Horo, Abinash Virk, Melanie D. Swift, John Halamka, Andrew D. Badley, A.J. Venkatakrishnan, Venky Soundararajan. Comparison of two highly-effective mRNA vaccines for COVID-19 during periods of Alpha and Delta variant prevalence. medRxiv 2021.08.06.21261707; doi: https://doi.org/10.11 01/2021.08.06.21261707
[116] Segerstrom SC, Miller GE. Psychological stress and the human immune system: a meta-analytic study of 30 years of inquiry. *Psychol Bull.* 2004;130(4):601-630. doi:10.1037/0033-2909.130.4.601
[117] Cain DW, Cidlowski JA. Immune regulation by glucocorticoids. *Nat Rev Immunol.* 2017;17(4):233-247. doi:10.1038/nri.2017.1
[118] Billard MJ, Gruver AL, Sempowski GD. Acute endotoxin-induced thymic atrophy is characterized by intrathymic inflammatory and wound healing

responses. *PLoS One.* 2011;6(3):e17940. Published 2011 Mar 18. doi:10.1371/journal.pone.0017940

[119] Cohen S, Janicki-Deverts D, Doyle WJ, et al. Chronic stress, glucocorticoid receptor resistance, inflammation, and disease risk. *Proc Natl Acad Sci U S A.* 2012;109(16):5995-5999. doi:10.1073/pnas.1118355109

[120] Tenforde MW, Kim SS, Lindsell CJ, et al. Symptom Duration and Risk Factors for Delayed Return to Usual Health Among Outpatients with COVID-19 in a Multistate Health Care Systems Network - United States, March-June 2020. MMWR Morb Mortal Wkly Rep. 2020;69(30):993-998. Published 2020 Jul 31. doi:10.15585/mmwr.mm6930e1

[121] Martel J, Ko YF, Young JD, Ojcius DM. Could nasal nitric oxide help to mitigate the severity of COVID-19?. *Microbes Infect.* 2020;22(4-5):168-171. doi:10.1016/j.micinf.2020.05.002

[122] https://www.clevelandheartlab.com/blog/nurturing-nitric-oxide-heart-healthy-chemical-blood-vessels/

[123] Li Q, Morimoto K, Nakadai A, et al. Forest bathing enhances human natural killer activity and expression of anti-cancer proteins. *Int J Immunopathol Pharmacol.* 2007;20(2 Suppl 2):3-8. doi:10.1177/03946320070200S202

[124] Woo J, Lee CJ. Sleep-enhancing Effects of Phytoncide Via Behavioral, Electrophysiological, and Molecular Modeling Approaches. *Exp Neurobiol.* 2020;29(2):120-129. doi:10.5607/en20013

[125] Black DS, Slavich GM. Mindfulness meditation and the immune system: a systematic review of randomized controlled trials. *Ann N Y Acad Sci.* 2016;1373(1):13-24. doi:10.1111/nyas.12998

[126] Fell GL, Robinson KC, Mao J, Woolf CJ, Fisher DE. Skin β-endorphin mediates addiction to UV light. *Cell.* 2014;157(7):1527-1534. doi:10.1016/j.cell.2014.04.032

[127] Sarris J, Mischoulon D, Schweitzer I. Omega-3 for bipolar disorder: meta-analyses of use in mania and bipolar depression. *J Clin Psychiatry.* 2012;73(1):81-86.

doi:10.4088/JCP.10r06710

128 Coffin CS, Shaffer EA. The hot air and cold facts of dietary fibre. *Can J Gastroenterol.* 2006;20(4):255-256. doi:10.1155/2006/390953

129 Yalagala PCR, Sugasini D, Dasarathi S, Pahan K, Subbaiah PV. Dietary lysophosphatidylcholine-EPA enriches both EPA and DHA in the brain: potential treatment for depression. *J Lipid Res.* 2019;60(3):566-578. doi:10.1194/jlr.M090464

130 Burns-Whitmore B, Froyen E, Heskey C, Parker T, San Pablo G. Alpha-Linolenic and Linoleic Fatty Acids in the Vegan Diet: Do They Require Dietary Reference Intake/Adequate Intake Special Consideration?. *Nutrients.* 2019;11(10):2365. Published 2019 Oct 4. doi:10.3390/nu11102365

131 Jacques A, Chaaya N, Beecher K, Ali SA, Belmer A, Bartlett S. The impact of sugar consumption on stress driven, emotional and addictive behaviors. *Neurosci Biobehav Rev.* 2019;103:178-199. doi:10.1016/j.neubiorev.2019.05.021

132 Anderson RJ, Grigsby AB, Freedland KE, et al. Anxiety and poor glycemic control: a meta-analytic review of the literature. *Int J Psychiatry Med.* 2002;32(3):235-247. doi:10.2190/KLGD-4H8D-4RYL-TWQ8

133 DiNicolantonio JJ, O'Keefe JH, Wilson W. Subclinical magnesium deficiency: a principal driver of cardiovascular disease and a public health crisis [published correction appears in Open Heart. 2018 Apr 5;5(1):e000668corr1]. *Open Heart.* 2018;5(1):e000668. Published 2018 Jan 13. doi:10.1136/openhrt-2017-000668

134 Cazzola R, Della Porta M, Manoni M, Iotti S, Pinotti L, Maier JA. Going to the roots of reduced magnesium dietary intake: A tradeoff between climate changes and sources. *Heliyon.* 2020;6(11):e05390. Published 2020 Nov 3. doi:10.1016/j.heliyon.2020.e05390

135 Pickering G, Mazur A, Trousselard M, et al. Magnesium Status and Stress: The Vicious Circle Concept

Revisited. *Nutrients*. 2020;12(12):3672. Published 2020 Nov 28. doi:10.3390/nu12123672

[136] Rosanoff, A. (2012). Changing crop magnesium concentrations: impact on human health. Plant and Soil, 368(1-2), 139–153. doi:10.1007/s11104-012-1471-5

[137] Bennett JW, Klich M. Mycotoxins. Clin Microbiol Rev. 2003;16(3):497-516. doi:10.1128/cmr.16.3.497-516.2003

[138] Lovallo WR, Whitsett TL, al'Absi M, Sung BH, Vincent AS, Wilson MF. Caffeine stimulation of cortisol secretion across the waking hours in relation to caffeine intake levels. *Psychosom Med*. 2005;67(5):734-739. doi:10.1097/01.psy.0000181270.20036.06

[139] Loftfield E, Cornelis MC, Caporaso N, Yu K, Sinha R, Freedman N. Association of Coffee Drinking With Mortality by Genetic Variation in Caffeine Metabolism: Findings From the UK Biobank. *JAMA Intern Med*. 2018;178(8):1086–1097. doi:10.1001/jamainternmed.2018.2425

[140] Nieber K. The Impact of Coffee on Health. *Planta Med*. 2017;83(16):1256-1263. doi:10.1055/s-0043-115007

[141] Patak P, Willenberg HS, Bornstein SR. Vitamin C is an important cofactor for both adrenal cortex and adrenal medulla. *Endocr Res*. 2004;30(4):871-875. doi:10.1081/erc-200044126

[142] Brody S, Preut R, Schommer K, Schürmeyer TH. A randomized controlled trial of high dose ascorbic acid for reduction of blood pressure, cortisol, and subjective responses to psychological stress. *Psychopharmacology (Berl)*. 2002;159(3):319-324. doi:10.1007/s00213-001-0929-6

[143] Kini P, Wong J, McInnis S, Gabana N, Brown JW. The effects of gratitude expression on neural activity. *Neuroimage*. 2016;128:1-10. doi:10.1016/j.neuroimage.2015.12.040

[144] Boggiss AL, Consedine NS, Brenton-Peters JM, Hofman PL, Serlachius AS. A systematic review of gratitude interventions: Effects on physical health and health behaviors. *J Psychosom Res*. 2020;135:110165.

doi:10.1016/j.jpsychores.2020.110165

145 Matvienko-Sikar K, Dockray S. Effects of a novel positive psychological intervention on prenatal stress and well-being: A pilot randomised controlled trial. *Women Birth.* 2017;30(2):e111-e118. doi:10.1016/j.wombi.2016.10.003

146 Mills PJ, Redwine L, Wilson K, et al. The Role of Gratitude in Spiritual Well-being in Asymptomatic Heart Failure Patients. *Spiritual Clin Pract (Wash D C).* 2015;2(1):5-17. doi:10.1037/scp0000050

147 Berk LS, Felten DL, Tan SA, Bittman BB, Westengard J. Modulation of neuroimmune parameters during the eustress of humor-associated mirthful laughter. *Altern Ther Health Med.* 2001;7(2):62-76

148 Bruce LD, Wu JS, Lustig SL, Russell DW, Nemecek DA. Loneliness in the United States: A 2018 National Panel Survey of Demographic, Structural, Cognitive, and Behavioral Characteristics. *Am J Health Promot.* 2019;33(8):1123-1133. doi:10.1177/0890117119856551

149 Malcolm M, Frost H, Cowie J. Loneliness and social isolation causal association with health-related lifestyle risk in older adults: a systematic review and meta-analysis protocol. *Syst Rev.* 2019;8(1):48. Published 2019 Feb 7. doi:10.1186/s13643-019-0968-x

150 Bhaskar S, Hemavathy D, Prasad S. Prevalence of chronic insomnia in adult patients and its correlation with medical comorbidities. *J Family Med Prim Care.* 2016;5(4):780-784. doi:10.4103/2249-4863.201153

151 Yazdi Z, Sadeghniiat-Haghighi K, Loukzadeh Z, Elmizadeh K, Abbasi M. Prevalence of Sleep Disorders and Their Impacts on Occupational Performance: A Comparison between Shift Workers and Nonshift Workers. Sleep Disord. 2014;2014:870320. doi:10.1155/2014/870320

152 Knutson KL, Ryden AM, Mander VA, Van Cauter E. Role of sleep duration and quality in the risk and severity of type 2 diabetes mellitus. Arch Intern

Med 2006;166:1768–1764.

[153] Kasasbeh E, Chi DS, Krishnaswamy G. Inflammatory aspects of sleep apnea and their cardiovascular consequences. South Med J 2006;99:58–67.

[154] Zimmerman M, McGlinchey JB, Young D, Chelminski I. Diagnosing major depressive disorder I: A psychometric evaluation of the DSM-IV symptom criteria. J Nerv Ment Dis 2006;194:158–163.

[155] Taheri S. The link between short sleep duration and obesity: We should recommend more sleep to prevent obesity. Arch Dis Child 2006;91:881–884.

[156] Besedovsky L, Lange T, Haack M. The Sleep-Immune Crosstalk in Health and Disease. *Physiol Rev.* 2019;99(3):1325-1380. doi:10.1152/physrev.00010.2018

[157] Huang B, Niu Y, Zhao W, Bao P, Li D. Reduced Sleep in the Week Prior to Diagnosis of COVID-19 is Associated with the Severity of COVID-19. *Nat Sci Sleep.* 2020;12:999-1007. Published 2020 Nov 12. doi:10.2147/NSS.S263488

[158] Kim H, Hegde S, LaFiura C, et alCOVID-19 illness in relation to sleep and burnoutBMJ Nutrition, Prevention & Health 2021;bmjnph-2021-000228. doi: 10.1136/bmjnph-2021-000228

[159] Grifoni A, Weiskopf D, Ramirez SI, et al. Targets of T Cell Responses to SARS-CoV-2 Coronavirus in Humans with COVID-19 Disease and Unexposed Individuals. *Cell.* 2020;181(7):1489-1501.e15. doi:10.1016/j.cell.2020.05.015

[160] Pouteau E, Kabir-Ahmadi M, Noah L, et al. Superiority of magnesium and vitamin B6 over magnesium alone on severe stress in healthy adults with low magnesemia: A randomized, single-blind clinical trial. *PLoS One.* 2018;13(12):e0208454. Published 2018 Dec 18. doi:10.1371/journal.pone.0208454

[161] Yamadera, W., Inagawa, K., Chiba, S. et al. Glycine ingestion improves subjective sleep quality in human volunteers, correlating with polysomnographic changes. Sleep Biol. Rhythms 5, 126–131 (2007).

https://doi.org/10.1111/j.1479-8425.2007.00262.x
162 Razak MA, Begum PS, Viswanath B, Rajagopal S. Multifarious Beneficial Effect of Nonessential Amino Acid, Glycine: A Review. Oxid Med Cell Longev. 2017;2017:1716701. doi:10.1155/2017/1716701
163 Kawai, N., Sakai, N., Okuro, M. et al. The Sleep-Promoting and Hypothermic Effects of Glycine are Mediated by NMDA Receptors in the Suprachiasmatic Nucleus. Neuropsychopharmacol 40, 1405–1416 (2015). https://doi.org/10.1038/npp.2014.326
164 Song CH, Jung JH, Oh JS, et al. Effects of Theanine on the Release of Brain Alpha Wave in Adult Males. *Korean J Nutr.* 2003;36(9):918-923.
165 Lyon MR, Kapoor MP, Juneja LR. The effects of L-theanine (Suntheanine®) on objective sleep quality in boys with attention deficit hyperactivity disorder (ADHD): a randomized, double-blind, placebo-controlled clinical trial. *Altern Med Rev.* 2011;16(4):348-354.
166 Kimura K, Ozeki M, Juneja LR, Ohira H. L-Theanine reduces psychological and physiological stress responses. *Biol Psychol.* 2007;74(1):39-45. doi:10.1016/j.biopsycho.2006.06.006
167 Kimura K, Ozeki M, Juneja LR, Ohira H. L-Theanine reduces psychological and physiological stress responses. *Biol Psychol.* 2007;74(1):39-45. doi:10.1016/j.biopsycho.2006.06.006
168 Mead MN. Benefits of sunlight: a bright spot for human health [published correction appears in Environ Health Perspect. 2008 May;116(5):A197]. *Environ Health Perspect.* 2008;116(4):A160-A167. doi:10.1289/ehp.116-a160
169 Majid MS, Ahmad HS, Bizhan H, Hosein HZM, Mohammad A. The effect of vitamin D supplement on the score and quality of sleep in 20-50 year-old people with sleep disorders compared with control group. Nutr Neurosci. 2018;21(7):511-519. doi:10.1080/1028415X.2017.1317395

[170] Viola H, Wasowski C, Levi de Stein M, et al. Apigenin, a component of Matricaria recutita flowers, is a central benzodiazepine receptors-ligand with anxiolytic effects. *Planta Med*. 1995;61(3):213-216. doi:10.1055/s-2006-958058

[171] Amsterdam JD, Shults J, Soeller I, Mao JJ, Rockwell K, Newberg AB. Chamomile (Matricaria recutita) may provide antidepressant activity in anxious, depressed humans: an exploratory study. *Altern Ther Health Med*. 2012;18(5):44-49.

[172] Hieu TH, Dibas M, Surya Dila KA, et al. Therapeutic efficacy and safety of chamomile for state anxiety, generalized anxiety disorder, insomnia, and sleep quality: A systematic review and meta-analysis of randomized trials and quasi-randomized trials. *Phytother Res*. 2019;33(6):1604-1615. doi:10.1002/ptr.6349

[173] Afaghi A, O'Connor H, Chow CM. High-glycemic-index carbohydrate meals shorten sleep onset [published correction appears in Am J Clin Nutr. 2007 Sep;86(3):809]. *Am J Clin Nutr*. 2007;85(2):426-430. doi:10.1093/ajcn/85.2.426

[174] Ayres, J.S. A metabolic handbook for the COVID-19 pandemic. Nat Metab 2, 572–585 (2020). https://doi.org/10.1038/s42255-020-0237-2

[175] Araújo J, Cai J, Stevens J. Prevalence of Optimal Metabolic Health in American Adults: National Health and Nutrition Examination Survey 2009-2016. Metab Syndr Relat Disord. 2019;17(1):46-52. doi:10.1089/met.2018.0105

[176] Clinical Guidelines on the Identification, Evaluation, and Treatment of Overweight and Obesity in Adults.

[177] Han TS, Lean ME. A clinical perspective of obesity, metabolic syndrome and cardiovascular disease. JRSM Cardiovasc Dis. 2016;5:2048004016633371. Published 2016 Feb 25. doi:10.1177/2048004016633371

[178] Bhaskaran K, Douglas I, Forbes H, dos-Santos-Silva I, Leon DA, Smeeth L. Body-mass index and risk of 22

specific cancers: a population-based cohort study of 5•24 million UK adults. Lancet. 2014 Aug 30;384(9945):755-65. doi: 10.1016/S0140-6736(14)60892-8. Epub 2014 Aug 13.

[179] Luppino, Floriana S., et al. "Overweight, obesity, and depression: a systematic review and meta-analysis of longitudinal studies." Archives of general psychiatry 67.3 (2010): 220-229.

[180] NHLBI. 2013. Managing Overweight and Obesity in Adults: Systematic Evidence Review from the Obesity Expert Panel

[181] Calvin C. Chan et al, Type I interferon sensing unlocks dormant adipocyte inflammatory potential, *Nature Communications* (2020).

[182] Craig M. Hales, M.D., Margaret D. Carroll, M.S.P.H., Cheryl D. Fryar, M.S.P.H., and Cynthia L. Ogden, Ph.D. Prevalence of Obesity and Severe Obesity Among Adults: United States, 2017–2018. NCHS Data Brief. No. 360. February 2020

[183] Edwards DA, Ausiello D, Salzman J, et al. Exhaled aerosol increases with COVID-19 infection, age, and obesity [published correction appears in Proc Natl Acad Sci U S A. 2021 Jul 6;118(27):]. Proc Natl Acad Sci U S A. 2021;118(8):e2021830118. doi:10.1073/pnas.2021830118

[184] Clemente JC, Ursell LK, Parfrey LW, Knight R. The impact of the gut microbiota on human health: an integrative view. *Cell*. 2012;148(6):1258-1270. doi:10.1016/j.cell.2012.01.035

[185] Sekirov I, Russell SL, Antunes LC, Finlay BB. Gut microbiota in health and disease. Physiol Rev. 2010;90(3):859-904. doi:10.1152/physrev.00045.2009

[186] Wilks J, Beilinson H, Golovkina TV. Dual role of commensal bacteria in viral infections. *Immunol Rev.* 2013;255(1):222-229. doi:10.1111/imr.12097

[187] Ichinohe T, Pang IK, Kumamoto Y, et al. Microbiota regulates immune defense against respiratory tract influenza A virus infection. *Proc Natl Acad Sci U S A.* 2011;108(13):5354-5359. doi:10.1073/pnas.1019378108

[188] Robinson CM, Pfeiffer JK. Viruses and the Microbiota. Annu Rev Virol. 2014;1:55-69. doi:10.1146/annurev-virology-031413-085550

[189] Channappanavar R, Fehr AR, Vijay R, et al. Dysregulated Type I Interferon and Inflammatory Monocyte-Macrophage Responses Cause Lethal Pneumonia in SARS-CoV-Infected Mice. Cell Host Microbe. 2016;19(2):181-193. doi:10.1016/j.chom.2016.01.007

[190] Zhang D, Li S, Wang N, Tan HY, Zhang Z, Feng Y. The Cross-Talk Between Gut Microbiota and Lungs in Common Lung Diseases. Front Microbiol. 2020;11:301. Published 2020 Feb 25. doi:10.3389/fmicb.2020.00301

[191] van der Lelie D, Taghavi S. COVID-19 and the Gut Microbiome: More than a Gut Feeling. *mSystems*. 2020;5(4):e00453-20. Published 2020 Jul 21. doi:10.1128/mSystems.00453-20

[192] Skalski JH, et al. Expansion of commensal fungus Wallemia mellicola in the gastrointestinal mycobiota enhances the severity of allergic airway disease in mice. PLOS Pathogens. 2018;20:e1007260.

[193] Demirci M, Tokman HB, Uysal HK, et al. Reduced Akkermansia muciniphila and Faecalibacterium prausnitzii levels in the gut microbiota of children with allergic asthma. *Allergol Immunopathol (Madr)*. 2019;47(4):365-371. doi:10.1016/j.aller.2018.12.009

[194] Tay MZ, Poh CM, Rénia L, MacAry PA, Ng LFP. The trinity of COVID-19: immunity, inflammation and intervention. Nat Rev Immunol. 2020;20(6):363-374. doi:10.1038/s41577-020-0311-8

[195] Yeoh YK, Zuo T, Lui GC, et al. Gut microbiota composition reflects disease severity and dysfunctional immune responses in patients with COVID-19. Gut. 2021;70(4):698-706. doi:10.1136/gutjnl-2020-323020

[196] Michael I McBurney, Cindy Davis, Claire M Fraser, Barbara O Schneeman, Curtis Huttenhower, Kristin Verbeke, Jens Walter, Marie E Latulippe, Establishing

What Constitutes a Healthy Human Gut Microbiome: State of the Science, Regulatory Considerations, and Future Directions, *The Journal of Nutrition*, Volume 149, Issue 11, November 2019, Pages 1882–1895, https://doi.org/10.1093/jn/nxz154

[197] Gosby AK, Conigrave AD, Lau NS, et al. Testing protein leverage in lean humans: a randomised controlled experimental study. PLoS One. 2011;6(10):e25929. doi:10.1371/journal.pone.0025929

[198] P.A. Lofgren. Meat, Poultry, and Meat Products: Nutritional Value. Editor(s): Benjamin Caballero. Encyclopedia of Human Nutrition (Third Edition). Academic Press. 2013. Pages 160-167. ISBN 9780123848857. https://doi.org/10.1016/B978-0-12-375083-9.00184-7.

[199] Maillot M, Darmon N, Darmon M, Lafay L, Drewnowski A. Nutrient-dense food groups have high energy costs: an econometric approach to nutrient profiling. *J Nutr*. 2007;137(7):1815-1820. doi:10.1093/jn/137.7.1815

[200] Ben-Dor M, Sirtoli R, Barkai R. The evolution of the human trophic level during the Pleistocene [published online ahead of print, 2021 Mar 5]. *Am J Phys Anthropol*. 2021;10.1002/ajpa.24247. doi:10.1002/ajpa.24247

[201] Neu J, Rushing J. Cesarean versus vaginal delivery: long-term infant outcomes and the hygiene hypothesis. Clin Perinatol. 2011;38(2):321-331. doi:10.1016/j.clp.2011.03.008

[202] Eggesbø M, Botten G, Stigum H, Nafstad P, Magnus P. Is delivery by cesarean section a risk factor for food allergy?. *J Allergy Clin Immunol*. 2003;112(2):420-426. doi:10.1067/mai.2003.1610

[203] Laubereau B, Filipiak-Pittroff B, von Berg A, et al. Caesarean section and gastrointestinal symptoms, atopic dermatitis, and sensitisation during the first year of life. Arch Dis Child. 2004;89(11):993-997. doi:10.1136/adc.2003.043265

204 Yang XT, Zhang WR, Tian ZC, et al. Depressive severity associated with cesarean section in young depressed individuals. Chin Med J (Engl). 2019;132(15):1883-1884. doi:10.1097/CM9.0000000000000326

205 Burton R, Sheron N. No level of alcohol consumption improves health. Lancet. 2018;392(10152):987-988. doi:10.1016/S0140-6736(18)31571-X

206 Simou E, Leonardi-Bee J, Britton J. The Effect of Alcohol Consumption on the Risk of ARDS: A Systematic Review and Meta-Analysis. Chest. 2018;154(1):58-68. doi:10.1016/j.chest.2017.11.041

207 Rehm J, Room R, Graham K, Monteiro M, Gmel G, Sempos CT. The relationship of average volume of alcohol consumption and patterns of drinking to burden of disease: an overview. Addiction. 2003;98(9):1209-1228. doi:10.1046/j.1360-0443.2003.00467.x

208 Veronese N, Watutantrige-Fernando S, Luchini C, et al. Effect of magnesium supplementation on glucose metabolism in people with or at risk of diabetes: a systematic review and meta-analysis of double-blind randomized controlled trials [published correction appears in Eur J Clin Nutr. 2016 Dec;70(12):1463]. Eur J Clin Nutr. 2016;70(12):1354-1359. doi:10.1038/ejcn.2016.154

209 Simental-Mendía LE, Sahebkar A, Rodríguez-Morán M, Guerrero-Romero F. A systematic review and meta-analysis of randomized controlled trials on the effects of magnesium supplementation on insulin sensitivity and glucose control. Pharmacol Res. 2016;111:272-282. doi:10.1016/j.phrs.2016.06.019

210 Nielsen FH. Effects of magnesium depletion on inflammation in chronic disease. Curr Opin Clin Nutr Metab Care. 2014;17(6):525-530. doi:10.1097/MCO.0000000000000093

211 Luan YY, Yao YM. The Clinical Significance and Potential Role of C-Reactive Protein in Chronic Inflammatory and Neurodegenerative Diseases. Front

Immunol. 2018;9:1302. Published 2018 Jun 7. doi:10.3389/fimmu.2018.01302

212 Hariyanto TI, Japar KV, Kwenandar F, et al. Inflammatory and hematologic markers as predictors of severe outcomes in COVID-19 infection: A systematic review and meta-analysis. *Am J Emerg Med.* 2021;41:110-119. doi:10.1016/j.ajem.2020.12.076

213 Chaigne-Delalande B, Li FY, O'Connor GM, et al. Mg2+ regulates cytotoxic functions of NK and CD8 T cells in chronic EBV infection through NKG2D. Science. 2013;341(6142):186-191. doi:10.1126/science.1240094

214 Jafar N, Edriss H, Nugent K. The Effect of Short-Term Hyperglycemia on the Innate Immune System. *Am J Med Sci.* 2016;351(2):201-211. doi:10.1016/j.amjms.2015.11.011

215 Tsujimoto T, Kajio H, Sugiyama T. Association between hyperinsulinemia and increased risk of cancer death in nonobese and obese people: A population-based observational study. Int J Cancer. 2017;141(1):102-111. doi:10.1002/ijc.30729

216 Feskens EJ, Kromhout D. Hyperinsulinemia, risk factors, and coronary heart disease. The Zutphen Elderly Study. Arterioscler Thromb. 1994 Oct;14(10):1641-7. doi: 10.1161/01.atv.14.10.1641. PMID: 7918315.

217 Cooper ID, Crofts CAP, DiNicolantonio JJ, et al. Relationships between hyperinsulinaemia, magnesium, vitamin D, thrombosis and COVID-19: rationale for clinical management. Open Heart. 2020;7(2):e001356. doi:10.1136/openhrt-2020-001356

218 Slavin J. Fiber and prebiotics: mechanisms and health benefits. *Nutrients.* 2013;5(4):1417-1435. Published 2013 Apr 22. doi:10.3390/nu5041417

219 Jardou M, Lawson R. Supportive therapy during COVID-19: The proposed mechanism of short-chain fatty acids to prevent cytokine storm and multi-organ failure. *Med Hypotheses.* 2021;154:110661. doi:10.1016/j.mehy.2021.110661

220 Trompette A, Gollwitzer ES, Pattaroni C, et al. Dietary

Fiber Confers Protection against Flu by Shaping Ly6c⁻ Patrolling Monocyte Hematopoiesis and CD8+ T Cell Metabolism. *Immunity*. 2018;48(5):992-1005.e8. doi:10.1016/j.immuni.2018.04.022

[221] Wastyk HC, Fragiadakis GK, Perelman D, et al. Gut-microbiota-targeted diets modulate human immune status. Cell. 2021;184(16):4137-4153.e14. doi:10.1016/j.cell.2021.06.019

[222] Chen LYC, Hoiland RL, Stukas S, Wellington CL, Sekhon MS. Assessing the importance of interleukin-6 in COVID-19. *Lancet Respir Med*. 2021;9(2):e13. doi:10.1016/S2213-2600(20)30600-7

[223] Patel RH, Mohiuddin SS. Biochemistry, Histamine. [Updated 2021 May 9]. In: StatPearls [Internet]. Treasure Island (FL): StatPearls Publishing; 2021 Jan-. Available from: https://www.ncbi.nlm.nih.gov/books/NBK557790/

[224] Eldanasory OA, Eljaaly K, Memish ZA, Al-Tawfiq JA. Histamine release theory and roles of antihistamine in the treatment of cytokines storm of COVID-19. Travel Med Infect Dis. 2020;37:101874. doi:10.1016/j.tmaid.2020.101874

[225] Kempuraj D, Selvakumar GP, Ahmed ME, et al. COVID-19, Mast Cells, Cytokine Storm, Psychological Stress, and Neuroinflammation. Neuroscientist. 2020;26(5-6):402-414. doi:10.1177/1073858420941476

[226] Afrin LB, Weinstock LB, Molderings GJ. Covid-19 hyperinflammation and post-Covid-19 illness may be rooted in mast cell activation syndrome. Int J Infect Dis. 2020;100:327-332. doi:10.1016/j.ijid.2020.09.016

[227] Mura C, Preissner S, Nahles S, Heiland M, Bourne PE, Preissner R. Real-world evidence for improved outcomes with histamine antagonists and aspirin in 22,560 COVID-19 patients. Signal Transduct Target Ther. 2021;6(1):267. Published 2021 Jul 14. doi:10.1038/s41392-021-00689-y

[228] Maintz L, Yu CF, Rodríguez E, et al. Association of single nucleotide polymorphisms in the diamine oxidase

gene with diamine oxidase serum activities. Allergy. 2011;66(7):893-902. doi:10.1111/j.1398-9995.2011.02548.x

229 Kritas SK, Gallenga CE, D Ovidio C, et al. Impact of mold on mast cell-cytokine immune response. J Biol Regul Homeost Agents. 2018;32(4):763-768.

230 Luttrell MJ, Halliwill JR. The Intriguing Role of Histamine in Exercise Responses. Exerc Sport Sci Rev. 2017;45(1):16-23. doi:10.1249/JES.0000000000000093

231 Carr AC, Maggini S. Vitamin C and Immune Function. Nutrients. 2017;9(11):1211. Published 2017 Nov 3. doi:10.3390/nu9111211

232 Saeedi-Boroujeni A, Mahmoudian-Sani MR. Anti-inflammatory potential of Quercetin in COVID-19 treatment. J Inflamm (Lond). 2021;18(1):3. Published 2021 Jan 28. doi:10.1186/s12950-021-00268-6

233 Dabbagh-Bazarbachi H, Clergeaud G, Quesada IM, Ortiz M, O'Sullivan CK, Fernández-Larrea JB. Zinc ionophore activity of quercetin and epigallocatechin-gallate: from Hepa 1-6 cells to a liposome model. J Agric Food Chem. 2014;62(32):8085-8093. doi:10.1021/jf5014633

234 DiNicolantonio JJ, O'Keefe JH. Omega-6 vegetable oils as a driver of coronary heart disease: the oxidized linoleic acid hypothesis. Open Heart. 2018;5(2):e000898. Published 2018 Sep 26. doi:10.1136/openhrt-2018-000898

235 Perumalla Venkata R, Subramanyam R. Evaluation of the deleterious health effects of consumption of repeatedly heated vegetable oil. Toxicol Rep. 2016;3:636-643. Published 2016 Aug 16. doi:10.1016/j.toxrep.2016.08.003

236 DiNicolantonio JJ, O'Keefe JH. Importance of maintaining a low omega-6/omega-3 ratio for reducing inflammation. *Open Heart*. 2018;5(2):e000946. Published 2018 Nov 26. doi:10.1136/openhrt-2018-000946

237 Russo GL. Dietary n-6 and n-3 polyunsaturated fatty acids: from biochemistry to clinical implications in cardiovascular prevention. Biochem Pharmacol. 2009;77(6):937-946. doi:10.1016/j.bcp.2008.10.020

238 Simopoulos AP. Evolutionary aspects of diet, the omega-6/omega-3 ratio and genetic variation: nutritional implications for chronic diseases. Biomed Pharmacother. 2006;60(9):502-507. doi:10.1016/j.biopha.2006.07.080

239 Hooper L, Al-Khudairy L, Abdelhamid AS, et al. Omega-6 fats for the primary and secondary prevention of cardiovascular disease. Cochrane Database Syst Rev. 2018;11(11):CD011094. Published 2018 Nov 29. doi:10.1002/14651858.CD011094.pub4

240 Wang DD, Li Y, Chiuve SE, et al. Association of Specific Dietary Fats With Total and Cause-Specific Mortality. JAMA Intern Med. 2016;176(8):1134-1145. doi:10.1001/jamainternmed.2016.2417

241 Siri-Tarino PW, Sun Q, Hu FB, Krauss RM. Meta-analysis of prospective cohort studies evaluating the association of saturated fat with cardiovascular disease. Am J Clin Nutr. 2010;91(3):535-546. doi:10.3945/ajcn.2009.27725

242 de Souza Russell J, Mente Andrew, Maroleanu Adriana, Cozma Adrian I, Ha Vanessa, Kishibe Teruko et al. Intake of saturated and trans unsaturated fatty acids and risk of all cause mortality, cardiovascular disease, and type 2 diabetes: systematic review and meta-analysis of observational studies BMJ 2015; 351 :h3978

243 Zhu Y, Bo Y, Liu Y. Dietary total fat, fatty acids intake, and risk of cardiovascular disease: a dose-response meta-analysis of cohort studies. *Lipids Health Dis.* 2019;18(1):91. Published 2019 Apr 6. doi:10.1186/s12944-019-1035-2

244 Kang ZQ, Yang Y, Xiao B. Dietary saturated fat intake and risk of stroke: Systematic review and dose-response meta-analysis of prospective cohort studies. Nutr Metab Cardiovasc Dis. 2020;30(2):179-189. doi:10.1016/j.numecd.2019.09.028

245 Ravnskov U, DiNicolantonio JJ, Harcombe Z, Kummerow FA, Okuyama H, Worm N. The questionable benefits of exchanging saturated fat with polyunsaturated

fat [published correction appears in Mayo Clin Proc. 2015 Apr;90(4):558]. Mayo Clin Proc. 2014;89(4):451-453. doi:10.1016/j.mayocp.2013.11.006

246 Astrup A, Magkos F, Bier DM, et al. Saturated Fats and Health: A Reassessment and Proposal for Food-Based Recommendations: JACC State-of-the-Art Review. J Am Coll Cardiol. 2020;76(7):844-857. doi:10.1016/j.jacc.2020.05.077

247 Fasano A. All disease begins in the (leaky) gut: role of zonulin-mediated gut permeability in the pathogenesis of some chronic inflammatory diseases. F1000Res. 2020;9:F1000 Faculty Rev-69. Published 2020 Jan 31. doi:10.12688/f1000research.20510.1

248 Sundqvist T, Lindström F, Magnusson KE, Sköldstam L, Stjernström I, Tagesson C. Influence of fasting on intestinal permeability and disease activity in patients with rheumatoid arthritis. Scand J Rheumatol. 1982;11(1):33-38. doi:10.3109/03009748209098111

249 Chen Q, Chen O, Martins IM, et al. Collagen peptides ameliorate intestinal epithelial barrier dysfunction in immunostimulatory Caco-2 cell monolayers via enhancing tight junctions. Food Funct. 2017;8(3):1144-1151. doi:10.1039/c6fo01347c

250 Dalla Pellegrina C, Perbellini O, Scupoli MT, et al. Effects of wheat germ agglutinin on human gastrointestinal epithelium: insights from an experimental model of immune/epithelial cell interaction. *Toxicol Appl Pharmacol.* 2009;237(2):146-153. doi:10.1016/j.taap.2009.03.012

251 Ovelgönne JH, Koninkx JF, Pusztai A, et al. Decreased levels of heat shock proteins in gut epithelial cells after exposure to plant lectins. *Gut.* 2000;46(5):679-687. doi:10.1136/gut.46.5.680

252 Vojdani A. Lectins, agglutinins, and their roles in autoimmune reactivities. *Altern Ther Health Med.* 2015;21 Suppl 1:46-51.

253 Freed DL. Do dietary lectins cause disease?. *BMJ.*

1999;318(7190):1023-1024.
doi:10.1136/bmj.318.7190.1023
[254] Smits SA, Leach J, Sonnenburg ED, et al. Seasonal cycling in the gut microbiome of the Hadza hunter-gatherers of Tanzania. *Science.* 2017;357(6353):802-806. doi:10.1126/science.aan4834
[255] Kalafati M, Jamurtas AZ, Nikolaidis MG, et al. Ergogenic and antioxidant effects of spirulina supplementation in humans. *Med Sci Sports Exerc.* 2010;42(1):142-151. doi:10.1249/MSS.0b013e3181ac7a45
[256] Moradi S, Ziaei R, Foshati S, Mohammadi H, Nachvak SM, Rouhani MH. Effects of Spirulina supplementation on obesity: A systematic review and meta-analysis of randomized clinical trials. *Complement Ther Med.* 2019;47:102211. doi:10.1016/j.ctim.2019.102211
[257] Cingi C, Conk-Dalay M, Cakli H, Bal C. The effects of spirulina on allergic rhinitis. *Eur Arch Otorhinolaryngol.* 2008;265(10):1219-1223. doi:10.1007/s00405-008-0642-8
[258] Bhatt A, Arora P, Prajapati SK. Can Algal Derived Bioactive Metabolites Serve as Potential Therapeutics for the Treatment of SARS-CoV-2 Like Viral Infection?. *Front Microbiol.* 2020;11:596374. Published 2020 Nov 11. doi:10.3389/fmicb.2020.596374
[259] Ratha SK, Renuka N, Rawat I, Bux F. Prospective options of algae-derived nutraceuticals as supplements to combat COVID-19 and human coronavirus diseases. *Nutrition.* 2021;83:111089. doi:10.1016/j.nut.2020.111089
[260] Rueda-Ruzafa L, Cruz F, Roman P, Cardona D. Gut microbiota and neurological effects of glyphosate. *Neurotoxicology.* 2019;75:1-8. doi:10.1016/j.neuro.2019.08.006
[261] Shehata AA, Schrödl W, Aldin AA, Hafez HM, Krüger M. The effect of glyphosate on potential pathogens and beneficial members of poultry microbiota in vitro. *Curr Microbiol.* 2013;66(4):350-358. doi:10.1007/s00284-012-0277-2

262 Domínguez-Díaz C, García-Orozco A, Riera-Leal A, Padilla-Arellano JR, Fafutis-Morris M. Microbiota and Its Role on Viral Evasion: Is It With Us or Against Us?. *Front Cell Infect Microbiol*. 2019;9:256. Published 2019 Jul 18. doi:10.3389/fcimb.2019.00256

263 Zhang L, Rana I, Shaffer RM, Taioli E, Sheppard L. Exposure to glyphosate-based herbicides and risk for non-Hodgkin lymphoma: A meta-analysis and supporting evidence. Mutat Res Rev Mutat Res. 2019;781:186-206. doi:10.1016/j.mrrev.2019.02.001

264 Rana I, Taioli E, Zhang L. Weeding out inaccurate information on glyphosate-based herbicides and risk of non-Hodgkin lymphoma. Environ Res. 2020;191:110140. doi:10.1016/j.envres.2020.110140

265 Meftaul IM, Venkateswarlu K, Dharmarajan R, et al. Controversies over human health and ecological impacts of glyphosate: Is it to be banned in modern agriculture?. *Environ Pollut*. 2020;263(Pt A):114372. doi:10.1016/j.envpol.2020.114372

266 Huxley RR, Ansary-Moghaddam A, Clifton P, Czernichow S, Parr CL, Woodward M. The impact of dietary and lifestyle risk factors on risk of colorectal cancer: a quantitative overview of the epidemiological evidence. *Int J Cancer*. 2009;125(1):171-180. doi:10.1002/ijc.24343

267 Madison A, Kiecolt-Glaser JK. Stress, depression, diet, and the gut microbiota: human-bacteria interactions at the core of psychoneuroimmunology and nutrition. Curr Opin Behav Sci. 2019;28:105-110. doi:10.1016/j.cobeha.2019.01.011

268 Brożyna AA, Hoffman RM, Slominski AT. Relevance of Vitamin D in Melanoma Development, Progression and Therapy. *Anticancer Res*. 2020;40(1):473-489. doi:10.21873/anticanres.13976

269 Brożyna AA, Hoffman RM, Slominski AT. Relevance of Vitamin D in Melanoma Development, Progression and Therapy. *Anticancer Res*. 2020;40(1):473-489.

doi:10.21873/anticanres.13976

[270] Field S, Newton-Bishop JA. Melanoma and vitamin D. *Mol Oncol*. 2011;5(2):197-214. doi:10.1016/j.molonc.2011.01.007

[271] Sarna M, Krzykawska-Serda M, Jakubowska M, Zadlo A, Urbanska K. Melanin presence inhibits melanoma cell spread in mice in a unique mechanical fashion. *Sci Rep*. 2019;9(1):9280. Published 2019 Jun 26. doi:10.1038/s41598-019-45643-9

[272] LaBerge GS, Duvall E, Grasmick Z, et al. Recent Advances in Studies of Skin Color and Skin Cancer. *Yale J Biol Med*. 2020;93(1):69-80. Published 2020 Mar 27.

[273] Holliman G, Lowe D, Cohen H, Felton S, Raj K. Ultraviolet Radiation-Induced Production of Nitric Oxide:A multi-cell and multi-donor analysis. Sci Rep. 2017;7(1):11105. Published 2017 Sep 11. doi:10.1038/s41598-017-11567-5

[274] Coleman JW. Nitric oxide in immunity and inflammation. Int Immunopharmacol. 2001;1(8):1397-1406. doi:10.1016/s1567-5769(01)00086-8

[275] Coleman JW. Nitric oxide in immunity and inflammation. Int Immunopharmacol. 2001;1(8):1397-1406. doi:10.1016/s1567-5769(01)00086-8

[276] Xu W, Zheng S, Dweik RA, Erzurum SC. Role of epithelial nitric oxide in airway viral infection. Free Radic Biol Med. 2006;41(1):19-28. doi:10.1016/j.freeradbiomed.2006.01.037

[277] Chowdhury R, Kunutsor S, Vitezova A, et al. Vitamin D and risk of cause specific death: systematic review and meta-analysis of observational cohort and randomised intervention studies. BMJ. 2014;348:g1903. Published 2014 Apr 1. doi:10.1136/bmj.g1903

[278] Forrest KY, Stuhldreher WL. Prevalence and correlates of vitamin D deficiency in US adults. Nutr Res. 2011;31(1):48-54. doi:10.1016/j.nutres.2010.12.001

[279] Chakhtoura M, Napoli N, El Hajj Fuleihan G. Commentary: Myths and facts on vitamin D amidst the

COVID-19 pandemic. *Metabolism.* 2020;109:154276. doi:10.1016/j.metabol.2020.154276

280 William B. Grant, Carol L. Wagner, Cedric F. Garland, Lorenz Borsche, Joseph Mercola. Vitamin D in the Prevention of COVID-19.

281 Hollis BW, Wagner CL, Howard CR, et al. Maternal Versus Infant Vitamin D Supplementation During Lactation: A Randomized Controlled Trial [published correction appears in Pediatrics. 2019 Jul;144(1):]. *Pediatrics.* 2015;136(4):625-634. doi:10.1542/peds.2015-1669

282 Wagner CL, Hollis BW. The implications of vitamin D status during pregnancy on mother and her developing child. Front Endocrinol (Lausanne) 2018; 9: 500.

283 Hollis BW, Johnson D, Hulsey TC, Ebeling M, Wagner CL. Vitamin D supplementation during pregnancy: double-blind, randomized clinical trial of safety and effectiveness. J Bone Miner Res 2011; 26: 2341-2357.

284 Mead MN. Benefits of sunlight: a bright spot for human health [published correction appears in Environ Health Perspect. 2008 May;116(5):A197]. Environ Health Perspect. 2008;116(4):A160-A167. doi:10.1289/ehp.116-a160

285 Parlak E, Ertürk A, Çağ Y, Sebin E, Gümüşdere M. The effect of inflammatory cytokines and the level of vitamin D on prognosis in Crimean-Congo hemorrhagic fever. Int J Clin Exp Med. 2015;8(10):18302-18310. Published 2015 Oct 15.

286 Dancer RC, Parekh D, Lax S, et al. Vitamin D deficiency contributes directly to the acute respiratory distress syndrome (ARDS). Thorax. 2015;70(7):617-624. doi:10.1136/thoraxjnl-2014-206680

287 Marik PE, Kory P, Varon J. Does vitamin D status impact mortality from SARS-CoV-2 infection? [published online ahead of print, 2020 Apr 29]. Med Drug Discov. 2020;6:100041. doi:10.1016/j.medidd.2020.100041

288 Martineau Adrian R, Jolliffe David A, Hooper Richard L, Greenberg Lauren, Aloia John F, Bergman Peter et

al. Vitamin D supplementation to prevent acute respiratory tract infections: systematic review and meta-analysis of individual participant data BMJ 2017; 356 :i6583

[289] McCullough PJ, Lehrer DS, Amend J. Daily oral dosing of vitamin D3 using 5000 TO 50,000 international units a day in long-term hospitalized patients: Insights from a seven year experience. *J Steroid Biochem Mol Biol.* 2019;189:228-239. doi:10.1016/j.jsbmb.2018.12.010

[290]

https://www.medrxiv.org/content/10.1101/2020.04.24.20075838v1

[291] Meltzer DO, Best TJ, Zhang H, Vokes T, Arora V, Solway J. Association of Vitamin D Deficiency and Treatment with COVID-19 Incidence. Preprint. *medRxiv.* 2020;2020.05.08.20095893. Published 2020 May 13. doi:10.1101/2020.05.08.20095893

[292]

https://www.medrxiv.org/content/10.1101/2020.04.08.20058578v4

[293] Castillo ME, Entrenas Costa LM, Vaquero Barrios JM, et al. "Effect of Calcifediol Treatment and best Available Therapy versus best Available Therapy on Intensive Care Unit Admission and Mortality Among Patients Hospitalized for COVID-19: A Pilot Randomized Clinical study" [published online ahead of print, 2020 Aug 29]. *J Steroid Biochem Mol Biol.* 2020;105751. doi:10.1016/j.jsbmb.2020.105751

[294] Kaufman HW, Niles JK, Kroll MH, Bi C, Holick MF. SARS-CoV-2 positivity rates associated with circulating 25-hydroxyvitamin D levels. PLoS One. 2020;15(9):e0239252. Published 2020 Sep 17. doi:10.1371/journal.pone.0239252

[295] Stroehlein JK, Wallqvist J, Iannizzi C, Mikolajewska A, Metzendorf M-I, Benstoem C, Meybohm P, Becker M, Skoetz N, Stegemann M, Piechotta V. Vitamin D supplementation for the treatment of COVID-19: a living systematic review. Cochrane Database of Systematic Reviews 2021, Issue 5.

Art. No.: CD015043. DOI: 10.1002/14651858.CD015043. Accessed 13 October 2021.

296 Murai IH, Fernandes AL, Sales LP, et al. Effect of a Single High Dose of Vitamin D3 on Hospital Length of Stay in Patients With Moderate to Severe COVID-19: A Randomized Clinical Trial. *JAMA*. 2021;325(11):1053-1060. doi:10.1001/jama.2020.26848

297 Marium Ilahi, Laura AG Armas, Robert P Heaney, Pharmacokinetics of a single, large dose of cholecalciferol, The American Journal of Clinical Nutrition, Volume 87, Issue 3, March 2008, Pages 688–691, https://doi.org/10.1093/ajcn/87.3.688

298 Amrein K, Scherkl M, Hoffmann M, et al. Vitamin D deficiency 2.0: an update on the current status worldwide. *Eur J Clin Nutr*. 2020;74(11):1498-1513. doi:10.1038/s41430-020-0558-y

299 Lorenz Borsche, Bernd Glauner, Julian von Mendel. 2021. COVID-19 mortality risk correlates inversely with vitamin D3 status, and a mortality rate close to zero could theoretically be achieved at 50 ng/ml 25(OH)D3: Results of a systematic review and meta-analysis. 09.22.21263977; doi: https://doi.org/10.1101/2021.09.22.21263977

300 Patwardhan VG, Mughal ZM, Padidela R, Chiplonkar SA, Khadilkar VV, Khadilkar AV. Randomized Control Trial Assessing Impact of Increased Sunlight Exposure versus Vitamin D Supplementation on Lipid Profile in Indian Vitamin D Deficient Men. Indian J Endocrinol Metab. 2017;21(3):393-398. doi:10.4103/ijem.IJEM_9_17

301 Kent ST, Cushman M, Howard G, et al. Sunlight exposure and cardiovascular risk factors in the REGARDS study: a cross-sectional split-sample analysis. BMC Neurol. 2014;14:133. Published 2014 Jun 19. doi:10.1186/1471-2377-14-133

302 Moradi S, Shahdadian F, Mohammadi H, Rouhani MH. A comparison of the effect of supplementation and sunlight exposure on serum vitamin D and parathyroid

hormone: A systematic review and meta-analysis. Crit Rev Food Sci Nutr. 2020;60(11):1881-1889. doi:10.1080/10408398.2019.1611538

[303] Uwitonze AM, Razzaque MS. Role of Magnesium in Vitamin D Activation and Function. J Am Osteopath Assoc. 2018;118(3):181-189. doi:10.7556/jaoa.2018.037

[304] van Ballegooijen AJ, Pilz S, Tomaschitz A, Grübler MR, Verheyen N. The Synergistic Interplay between Vitamins D and K for Bone and Cardiovascular Health: A Narrative Review. Int J Endocrinol. 2017;2017:7454376. doi:10.1155/2017/7454376

[305] Anton S M Dofferhoff, M.D, Ianthe Piscaer, M.D, Leon J Schurgers, PhD, Margot P J Visser, M.D, Jody M W van den Ouweland, Ph.D, Pim A de Jong, M.D, Reinoud Gosens, Ph.D, Tilman M Hackeng, Ph.D, Henny van Daal, Petra Lux, Cecile Maassen, Esther G A Karssemeijer, M.D, Cees Vermeer, Ph.D, Emiel F M Wouters, M.D, Loes E M Kistemaker, Ph.D, Jona Walk, M.D, Rob Janssen, M.D, Reduced vitamin K status as a potentially modifiable risk factor of severe COVID-19, Clinical Infectious Diseases, , ciaa1258, https://doi.org/10.1093/cid/ciaa1258

[306] Saurat, J.-H. (2001). Skin, Sun, and Vitamin A: From Aging to Cancer. The Journal of Dermatology, 28(11), 595–598. doi:10.1111/j.1346-8138.2001.tb00040.x

[307] Heinrich U, Neukam K, Tronnier H, Sies H, Stahl W. Long-term ingestion of high flavanol cocoa provides photoprotection against UV-induced erythema and improves skin condition in women. J Nutr. 2006;136(6):1565-1569. doi:10.1093/jn/136.6.1565

[308] Ito N, Seki S, Ueda F. The Protective Role of Astaxanthin for UV-Induced Skin Deterioration in Healthy People-A Randomized, Double-Blind, Placebo-Controlled Trial. Nutrients. 2018;10(7):817. Published 2018 Jun 25. doi:10.3390/nu10070817

[309] Scheuer C, Pommergaard HC, Rosenberg J, Gögenur I. Melatonin's protective effect against UV radiation: a

systematic review of clinical and experimental studies. *Photodermatol Photoimmunol Photomed.* 2014;30(4):180-188. doi:10.1111/phpp.12080
310 https://www.cdc.gov/nceh/radiation/nonionizing_radiation.html
311 Zorach R. Glaser, Ph.D. LT, MSC, USNR. 1971. BIBLIOGPHY OF REPORTED BIOLOGICAL PHENOMENA ('EFFECTS') AND CLINICAL MANIFESTATIONS ATTRIBUrED TO MICROWAVE AND RADIO-FREQUENCY RADIATION. Project MF12.524.015-00043,Report No. 2 Naval Medical Research Institute National Naval Medical Center Bethesda, Maryland 20014, U.S.A.
312 WHO (World Health Organisation), "Electromagnetic hypersensitivity," in Proceedings of the International Workshop on EMF Hypersensitivity, Prague, Czech Republic, 2004.
313 Dr. Martin Pall. 2018. 5G: Great risk for EU, U.S. and International Health! Compelling Evidence for Eight Distinct Types of Great Harm Caused by Electromagnetic Field (EMF) Exposures and the Mechanism that Causes Them
314 Pall, ML. 2013. Electromagnetic fields act via activation of voltage-gated calcium channels to produce beneficial or adverse effects. J Cell Mol Med 17:958-965. doi: 10.1111/jcmm.12088.
315 Huss A, Egger M, Hug K, Huwiler-Müntener K, Röösli M. Source of funding and results of studies of health effects of mobile phone use: systematic review of experimental studies. Environ Health Perspect. 2007;115(1):1-4. doi:10.1289/ehp.9149
316 Hardell L. World Health Organization, radiofrequency radiation and health - a hard nut to crack (Review). Int J Oncol. 2017;51(2):405-413. doi:10.3892/ijo.2017.4046
317 https://bioinitiative.org/
318 National Toxicology Program. March 26–28, 2018.

Peer Review of the Draft NTP Technical Reports on Cell Phone Radiofrequency Radiation.
https://ntp.niehs.nih.gov/ntp/about_ntp/trpanel/2018/march/peerreview20180328_508.pdf
[319] Martin L. Pall, PhD. *5G: Great risk for EU, U.S. and International Health! Compelling Evidence for Eight Distinct Types of Great Harm Caused by Electromagnetic Field (EMF) Exposures and the Mechanism that Causes Them*
[320] Johansson O. Disturbance of the immune system by electromagnetic fields-A potentially underlying cause for cellular damage and tissue repair reduction which could lead to disease and impairment. *Pathophysiology.* 2009;16(2-3):157-177. doi:10.1016/j.pathophys.2009.03.004
[321] 1977. Effects of Nonionizing Electromagnetic Radiation. Translations on USSR Science and Technology. *Biomedical Sciences.*
[322] Lerchl A, Klose M, Grote K, et al. Tumor promotion by exposure to radiofrequency electromagnetic fields below exposure limits for humans. *Biochem Biophys Res Commun.* 2015;459(4):585-590. doi:10.1016/j.bbrc.2015.02.151
[323] Volkow ND, Tomasi D, Wang GJ, et al. Effects of cell phone radiofrequency signal exposure on brain glucose metabolism. *JAMA.* 2011;305(8):808-813. doi:10.1001/jama.2011.186
[324] Aldad, T., Gan, G., Gao, X. *et al.* Fetal Radiofrequency Radiation Exposure From 800-1900 Mhz-Rated Cellular Telephones Affects Neurodevelopment and Behavior in Mice. *Sci Rep* **2,** 312 (2012). https://doi.org/10.1038/srep00312
[325] Sonmez OF, Odaci E, Bas O, Kaplan S. Purkinje cell number decreases in the adult female rat cerebellum following exposure to 900 MHz electromagnetic field. *Brain Res.* 2010;1356:95-101. doi:10.1016/j.brainres.2010.07.103
[326] Salford LG, Brun AE, Eberhardt JL, Malmgren L, Persson BR. Nerve cell damage in mammalian brain after

exposure to microwaves from GSM mobile phones. *Environ Health Perspect.* 2003;111(7):881-A408. doi:10.1289/ehp.6039

327 Touyz RM. Magnesium supplementation as an adjuvant to synthetic calcium channel antagonists in the treatment of hypertension. Med Hypotheses. 1991;36(2):140-141. doi:10.1016/0306-9877(91)90256-x

328 Altun G, Kaplan S, Deniz OG, et al. Protective effects of melatonin and omega-3 on the hippocampus and the cerebellum of adult Wistar albino rats exposed to electromagnetic fields. J Microsc Ultrastruct. 2017;5(4):230-241. doi:10.1016/j.jmau.2017.05.006

329 Sepehrimanesh, M., Kazemipour, N., Saeb, M. *et al.* Proteomic analysis of continuous 900-MHz radiofrequency electromagnetic field exposure in testicular tissue: a rat model of human cell phone exposure. *Environ Sci Pollut Res* **24,** 13666–13673 (2017). https://doi.org/10.1007/s11356-017-8882-z

330 West JG, Kapoor NS, Liao SY, Chen JW, Bailey L, Nagourney RA. Multifocal Breast Cancer in Young Women with Prolonged Contact between Their Breasts and Their Cellular Phones. *Case Rep Med.* 2013;2013:354682. doi:10.1155/2013/354682

331 Sangun O, Dundar B, Darici H, Comlekci S, Doguc DK, Celik S. The effects of long-term exposure to a 2450 MHz electromagnetic field on growth and pubertal development in female Wistar rats. *Electromagn Biol Med.* 2015;34(1):63-71. doi:10.3109/15368378.2013.871619

332 Shahin S, Singh VP, Shukla RK, et al. 2.45 GHz microwave irradiation-induced oxidative stress affects implantation or pregnancy in mice, Mus musculus. *Appl Biochem Biotechnol.* 2013;169(5):1727-1751. doi:10.1007/s12010-012-0079-9

333 Oschman JL, Chevalier G, Brown R. The effects of grounding (earthing) on inflammation, the immune response, wound healing, and prevention and treatment of chronic inflammatory and autoimmune diseases. *J Inflamm*

Res. 2015;8:83-96. Published 2015 Mar 24.
doi:10.2147/JIR.S69656

334 Chevalier G, Patel S, Weiss L, Chopra D, Mills PJ. The Effects of Grounding (Earthing) on Bodyworkers' Pain and Overall Quality of Life: A Randomized Controlled Trial. *Explore (NY).* 2019;15(3):181-190.
doi:10.1016/j.explore.2018.10.001

335 Chevalier G, Sinatra ST, Oschman JL, Delany RM. Earthing (grounding) the human body reduces blood viscosity-a major factor in cardiovascular disease. *J Altern Complement Med.* 2013;19(2):102-110.
doi:10.1089/acm.2011.0820

336 Taco-Vasquez ED, Barrera F, Serrano-Duenas M, Jimenez E, Rocuts A, Riveros Perez E. Association between Blood Viscosity and Cardiovascular Risk Factors in Patients with Arterial Hypertension in a High Altitude Setting. *Cureus.* 2019;11(1):e3925. Published 2019 Jan 21.
doi:10.7759/cureus.3925

337 Maier CL, Truong AD, Auld SC, Polly DM, Tanksley CL, Duncan A. COVID-19-associated hyperviscosity: a link between inflammation and thrombophilia?. *Lancet.* 2020;395(10239):1758-1759. doi:10.1016/S0140-6736(20)31209-5

338 Colbey C, Cox AJ, Pyne DB, Zhang P, Cripps AW, West NP. Upper Respiratory Symptoms, Gut Health and Mucosal Immunity in Athletes. Sports Med. 2018;48(Suppl 1):65-77. doi:10.1007/s40279-017-0846-4

339 Cicchella A, Stefanelli C, Massaro M. Upper Respiratory Tract Infections in Sport and the Immune System Response. A Review. Biology (Basel). 2021;10(5):362. Published 2021 Apr 23.
doi:10.3390/biology10050362

340 Dubnov-Raz G, Livne N, Raz R, Cohen AH, Constantini NW. Vitamin D Supplementation and Physical Performance in Adolescent Swimmers. Int J Sport Nutr Exerc Metab. 2015;25(4):317-325.
doi:10.1123/ijsnem.2014-0180

341 Baek SS. Role of exercise on the brain. *J Exerc Rehabil.* 2016;12(5):380-385. Published 2016 Oct 31. doi:10.12965/jer.1632808.404

342 Chastin SFM, Abaraogu U, Bourgois JG, et al. Effects of Regular Physical Activity on the Immune System, Vaccination and Risk of Community-Acquired Infectious Disease in the General Population: Systematic Review and Meta-Analysis. Sports Med. 2021;51(8):1673-1686. doi:10.1007/s40279-021-01466-1

343 Vina J, Sanchis-Gomar F, Martinez-Bello V, Gomez-Cabrera MC. Exercise acts as a drug; the pharmacological benefits of exercise. *Br J Pharmacol.* 2012;167(1):1-12. doi:10.1111/j.1476-5381.2012.01970.x

344 Lee SW, Lee J, Moon SY, et al. Physical activity and the risk of SARS-CoV-2 infection, severe COVID-19 illness and COVID-19 related mortality in South Korea: a nationwide cohort study [published online ahead of print, 2021 Jul 22]. *Br J Sports Med.* 2021;bjsports-2021-104203. doi:10.1136/bjsports-2021-104203

345 Brawner CA, Ehrman JK, Bole S, et al. Inverse Relationship of Maximal Exercise Capacity to Hospitalization Secondary to Coronavirus Disease 2019. *Mayo Clin Proc.* 2021;96(1):32-39. doi:10.1016/j.mayocp.2020.10.003

346 Pontzer H, Wood BM, Raichlen DA. Hunter-gatherers as models in public health. *Obes Rev.* 2018;19 Suppl 1:24-35. doi:10.1111/obr.12785

347 Krzyścin JW, Guzikowski J, Rajewska-Więch B. Optimal vitamin D3 daily intake of 2000IU inferred from modeled solar exposure of ancestral humans in Northern Tanzania. *J Photochem Photobiol B.* 2016;159:101-105. doi:10.1016/j.jphotobiol.2016.03.029

348 Gando S. Microvascular thrombosis and multiple organ dysfunction syndrome. Crit Care Med. 2010;38(2 Suppl):S35-S42. doi:10.1097/CCM.0b013e3181c9e31d

349 Wu X, Nethery RC, Sabath BM, Braun D, Dominici F. Exposure to air pollution and COVID-19 mortality in the

United States: A nationwide cross-sectional study. Preprint. *medRxiv*. 2020;2020.04.05.20054502. Published 2020 Apr 7. doi:10.1101/2020.04.05.20054502

[350] Wu X, Nethery RC, Sabath MB, Braun D, Dominici F. Air pollution and COVID-19 mortality in the United States: Strengths and limitations of an ecological regression analysis. Sci Adv. 2020;6(45):eabd4049. Published 2020 Nov 4. doi:10.1126/sciadv.abd4049

[351] https://aqicn.org/city/usa/newyork/

[352] Setti L, Passarini F, De Gennaro G, et al. SARS-Cov-2RNA found on particulate matter of Bergamo in Northern Italy: First evidence. Environ Res. 2020;188:109754. doi:10.1016/j.envres.2020.109754

[353] O'Hearn M, Liu J, Cudhea F, Micha R, Mozaffarian D. Coronavirus Disease 2019 Hospitalizations Attributable to Cardiometabolic Conditions in the United States: A Comparative Risk Assessment Analysis [published online ahead of print, 2021 Feb 25]. *J Am Heart Assoc.* 2021;e019259. doi:10.1161/JAHA.120.019259

[354] Centers for Disease Control and Prevention. Weekly Updates by Select Demographic and Geographic Characteristics. Provisional Death Counts for Coronavirus Disease 2019 (COVID-19).

[355] Sustainable Agriculture Research & Education. "Rotations and Soil Organic Matter Levels." *SARE,* (n.d.) Retrieved March 13, 2019, from https://www.sare.org/Learning-Center/Books/Building-Soils-for-Better-Crops-3rd-Edition/Text-Version/Crop-Rotations/Rotations-and-Soil-Organic-Matter-Levels

[356] van Uhm DP. The Sixth Mass Extinction. The Illegal Wildlife Trade. 2016;15:17-32. Published 2016 Nov 16. doi:10.1007/978-3-319-42129-2_2

[357] Dirzo R, Young HS, Galetti M, Ceballos G, Isaac NJ, Collen B. Defaunation in the Anthropocene. Science. 2014;345(6195):401-406. doi:10.1126/science.1251817

[358] Ontl, Todd A. and Schulte, Lisa A. "Soil Carbon

Storage." *The Nature Education Knowledge Project,* 3(10):35 (2012). Retrieved March 13, 2019, from https://www.nature.com/scitable/knowledge/library/soil-carbon-storage-84223790

359 Gilpin W, Feldman MW, Aoki K. An ecocultural model predicts Neanderthal extinction through competition with modern humans. Proc Natl Acad Sci U S A. 2016;113(8):2134-2139. doi:10.1073/pnas.1524861113